OSAP.org

The Safest Dental Visit™

C0-BJY-378

OSHA & CDC Guidelines

OSAP Interact
Training System

Combining Safety with Infection Control for Dentistry

Name:

_____

Name and Address of Practice/School:

_____

_____

_____

_____

Disclaimer:

This workbook is intended to offer general guidelines to healthcare providers, students, and employers on infection control, hazard communication, waste management, employee training, and related topics. The information contained herein should not be construed as legal advice and may not be substituted for the legal advice of the healthcare provider's own legal counsel.

Users of the program are encouraged to maintain a membership in the Organization for Safety, Asepsis and Prevention (OSAP), as updates in regulations and other issues are provided monthly.

OSAP
3525 Piedmont Road, NE
Building 5, Ste. 300
Atlanta, GA 30305-1509

IBSN-13:978-0-9752519-3-5

Acknowledgments:

Authors

Kathy J. Eklund, RDH, MHP
Director of Occupational Health and Safety
The Forsyth Institute

Helene Bednarsh, BS, RDH, MPH
Director Ryan White Dental Program
Boston Public Health Commission

Christian O. Haaland, BS, MBA
President, Invision, Inc.

Reviewers: 6th Edition

Kathy J. Eklund, RDH MHP
Director of Occupational Health and Safety
The Forsyth Institute

Helene Bednarsh, BS, RDH, MPH
Director Ryan White Dental Program
Boston Public Health Commission

Chris H. Miller, PhD
Professor Emeritus of Microbiology
Executive Associate Dean Emeritus
Associate Dean Emeritus for Academic Affairs and for Graduate Education
Indiana University School of Dentistry

Ashley MacDermott, MPH, CHES
Director of Education
Organization for Safety, Asepsis and Prevention (OSAP)

Contents:

Notes:

- The pages in this book are numbered per chapter in the upper corners.
  For example:
  page 8 of course #1 is shown as **1 · 8**
  page 8 of course #2 is shown as **2 · 8**

- This course is not a substitute for recommendations from the CDC, regulations from OSHA, or requirements of state and local agencies.

- Portions of this text have been taken from the CDC *Guidelines for Infection Control in Dental Health-Care Settings - 2003*, the CDC *Summary of Infection Prevention Practices in Dental Settings: Basic Expectations for Safe Care*, the OSHA Bloodborne Pathogens Standard, and the Hazard Communication Standard.

Continuing Education Units Documentation

OSAP Interact Training   **Date Completed**

Use the following chart to document completion of each training module
as well as any additional infection control and safety training. Place a copy
of this training documentation in the employee's training record.

1. Introduction _____

2. Occupational Exposure _____

3. Personal Protection _____

4. A Practical Program for Exposure Control _____

5. Instrument Reprocessing _____

6. Product Selection _____

7. Written Procedures _____

8. Hazard Communication _____

9. Medical Waste Disposal _____

10. Pulling it all Together _____

Additional Training

Course/Seminar	Location	Instructor	Date Completed	Hours
_____	_____	_____	_____	_____
_____	_____	_____	_____	_____
_____	_____	_____	_____	_____
_____	_____	_____	_____	_____
_____	_____	_____	_____	_____
_____	_____	_____	_____	_____
_____	_____	_____	_____	_____
_____	_____	_____	_____	_____
_____	_____	_____	_____	_____
_____	_____	_____	_____	_____
_____	_____	_____	_____	_____
_____	_____	_____	_____	_____

Yearly Training Total: _____

What OSAP Can Do
FOR YOU

OSAP is an objective, truste[d] global resource for infectio[n] prevention & safety issue[s] questions, leadersh[ip] contacts, education, poli[cy] development, and servi[ces] supporting The Safest Dent[al] Visit[T]

THE VALUE OF **OSAP**

We advocate for the safe and infection-free delivery of oral healthcare.

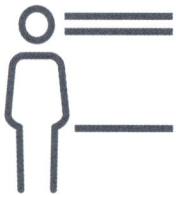

TRAIN

A leading provider of education that supports safe dental visits. Dental Infection Control Boot Camp™, Annual Conference, Webinars

CERTIFY

Certificate and Certification Program to elevate the individual's knowledge of dental infection control. Learn more at *DentalInfectionControl.org*

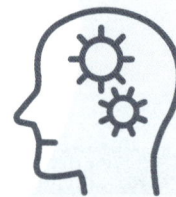

INFORM

Keeping the global dental community up to date on the latest in infection prevention: *Journal of Dental Infection Control and Safety*, InfoBites, ICIP (Infection Control In Practice), and more

OSAP .org
The Safest Dental Visit™

Objectives

Upon completion of this course, you will be able to:
1. Describe four principles of infection control.
2. Differentiate the roles of OSHA and CDC.

Focus

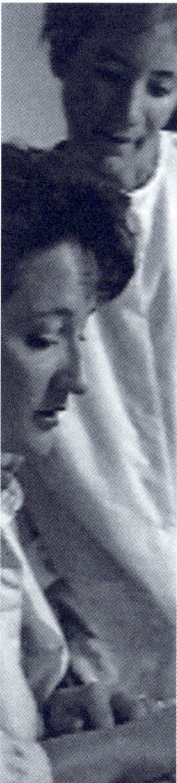

Every instrument you handle, every patient you deal with, and every piece of contaminated material you touch, has with it certain procedures that must be followed to protect you, your co-workers, and your patients. As this training system leads you, step-by-step, through a wide variety of information, you will – almost without knowing it – develop safe and practical working habits.

Your health and safety and that of the patients you serve are a major focus of public health advisors, the media, and the public. This focus defines how dentistry is practiced. "Quality care" has been expanded to include the health and safety considerations of both the patient and you: the healthcare worker.

These health and safety considerations, established by government guidelines and regulations, only appear to be complex and confusing. In fact, it is the interpretation of the many recommendations and requirements that can be difficult. This course makes understanding these recommendations easy, and is designed to train you to develop safe working habits through their practical application. In the process, the steps necessary to comply with government regulations are simplified. The bottom line is that these regulations exist with only one purpose in mind: to protect you.

In the day-to-day practice of dentistry, it is difficult to develop a comprehensive and practical training program including new office procedures that complies with all the standards, regulations, and requirements. Our approach is to address not only compliance with government regulations, but also to explain and demonstrate procedures so they will become part of your daily routine. This makes you an integral part of a safe office.

This program leads you through the process of learning how to be safe in the workplace in ten easy-to-understand lessons:

1. **Introduction - What Am I Getting Into?**
2. **Occupational Exposure - Why You Need to be Careful**
3. **Personal Protection - Barriers for Everyone**
4. **A Practical Program for Exposure Control - Your Daily Procedures**
5. **Instrument Reprocessing - Cleaning, Packaging, Sterilization**
6. **Product Selection - Cost Effective Product Selection**
7. **Written Procedures - Policies, Procedures, and Record-Keeping**
8. **Hazard Communication (HAZCOM) - The Hazard Communication Standard**
9. **Medical Waste Disposal - Handling, Packaging, Transport, and Records**
10. **Pulling it all Together - Integrated Office Management**

There are three sequential parts to each course: The information in the workbook, the one-on-one or group follow-up discussion, and the self-assessment documentation.

1. Workbook

Your workbook is designed to explain and reference a wide array of infection control and related health and safety issues. In each module, there are fill-in-the-blank questions designed to familiarize you with locations and procedures specific to your office and to aid in comprehension.

2. Discussion

Your office's Infection Control Coordinator and/or employer will discuss with you and clarify any aspect of the material presented, demonstrate any particular procedures used in your office, and show you the location of resources, equipment, and materials.

3. Documentation

After each course, there is a short self-assessment test to highlight the key points in each lesson and to evaluate your knowledge of your office's procedures. This signed test serves as your office's training record and must be kept in your personnel file for three years, to meet the US Department of Labor's Occupational Safety and Health Administration's (OSHA) training requirements.

Note:

You can complete step #1 above, either by yourself or as part of a group, and it is not necessary to have your Infection Control Coordinator/Dentist or Employer present. However, government regulations stipulate that ample time must be provided during training for discussion with one of them, which is step #2.

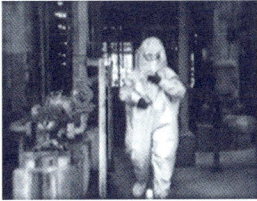

The US Department of Labor, by an act of Congress, created the Occupational Safety and Health Administration (OSHA) in 1970 for the sole purpose of protecting the health and safety of all workers. OSHA mandated, through its General Duty Clause that:

> **Each employer must "furnish to each of his employees, employment and a place of employment, which are free from recognized hazards that are causing or are likely to cause death or serious physical harm to his employees."**

OSHA's first enforcement efforts were in the manufacturing and mining industries, which were experiencing the greatest number of work-related injuries. These early general industry regulations were designed to control air quality, noise, hazardous chemicals and materials, building design, and access to employee records. It was not until 1987 that overall chemical safety was addressed in the Hazard Communication Standard *Title 29, Code of Federal Regulations (CFR) Part 1910.1200*, which requires that the hazards associated with the production, transportation, usage, storage, and disposal of chemicals be communicated to all employees. Chemicals are used every day in dental settings and some are hazardous. When hazardous chemicals are used in the workplace, the Hazard Communication Standard requires a hazard communication program. This program includes a written document that describes labeling containers of hazardous chemicals, use of safety data sheets (SDS) for hazardous chemicals, and staff training. Hazard Communication (HAZCOM) is covered in course #8.

Regulations for Healthcare Workers

Initially, there were no specific regulations included for the control of bloodborne infectious diseases in the healthcare environment, as there was no perception that healthcare workers were at significant risk. In the mid-1980's, OSHA recognized that healthcare workers are exposed to a variety of hazards, the most serious of which was the hepatitis B virus (HBV). A new vaccination became commercially available for preventing HBV infection in 1982, and voluntary guidelines were issued by OSHA in 1983 to encourage the vaccination's use. Additionally, a new threat emerged in a bloodborne virus, transmitted via body fluids in a manner similar to hepatitis B virus, and was identified as "human immunodeficiency virus" or HIV. This new virus was also a consideration in the issuing of suggested, voluntary guidelines, which, in effect, said nothing more than "be immunized" for HBV and use gloves and masks while treating patients.

Unfortunately these voluntary guidelines had no legal enforcement ability to protect healthcare workers, and consequently, in 1986, the government began to develop new mandatory standards. Proposed regulations for the new Occupational Exposure to Bloodborne Pathogens *29 CFR Part 1910.1030 (Bloodborne Pathogens Standard)* were issued in May, 1989 and finalized on December 6, 1991. When issuing the "Final Rule," OSHA's administrator said:

> **"Today we are providing full legal force to universal precautions — employers and employees must treat blood and certain body fluids as if infectious. Meeting these requirements is not optional. It's essential to prevent illness, chronic infection and even death." Universal precautions are now part of what CDC refers to as Standard Precautions.**

1970 · **OSHA Created**
1983 · **Voluntary Infection Control Standards Issued**
1986 · **Began to Develop New Bloodborne Standards**
1987 · **Hazard Communication Standard Issued**
1991 · **Final, Mandatory Bloodborne Pathogens Standard Issued**
1995 · **Dental Employer Obligations for Postexposure Management Defined**
2001 · **Bloodborne Pathogens Standard Revision**
2012 · **Hazard Communication Standard Revision**

CDC Recommendations for Healthcare Workers

The Centers for Disease Control and Prevention (CDC) is the foremost public health agency in the United States. It reviews current scientific information and based on that information, creates recommendations to protect the health of the population at large. CDC also tracks disease trends across the country and may serve as primary investigator when disease outbreaks threaten public health. Using the information it gathers, the agency develops methods for preventing or limiting the occurrence of all diseases.

Unlike OSHA, a regulatory agency that is only concerned with employees, CDC develops guidelines designed to protect workers and patients. The CDC developed four major principles to control the spread of infectious diseases from workers to patients, from patients to workers, and between patients.

Take action to stay healthy	Limit the spread of contamination
• **Get immunized**	• **Set up the operatory before starting treatment**
• **Report occupational injuries and exposures immediately**	• **Unit dose supplies**
• **Follow the advice of the medical care provider evaluating your occupational exposure**	• **Cover surfaces that will be contaminated**
	• **Minimize splashes and spatter**
• **Wash hands**	• **Properly dispose of all waste**

Avoid contacting blood/body fluids	Make objects safe for use
• **Wear gloves, protective clothing, and face and eye protection**	• **Monitor processes to make sure they're working as they should**
• **Handle sharps with care**	• **Dispose of single-use items**
• **Use safety devices as appropriate**	• **Follow appropriate instrument reprocessing (e.g., sterilization) for reusable items**
• **Use mechanical devices to clean instruments whenever possible**	• **Sharp devices with engineered safety measures**

Since the release of the Bloodborne Pathogens Standard, OSHA and the CDC have acknowledged that other biological hazards exist that may affect healthcare workers and their patients. Professional organizations such as the Organization for Safety, Asepsis and Prevention (OSAP), the American Dental Association (ADA), the American Dental Hygienists Association (ADHA), the American Dental Assisting Association (ADAA), and the Association for Professionals in Infection Control and Epidemiology (APIC), among others, have developed recommendations for safer workplaces. Specifically, there has been increased attention to hepatitis C, airborne diseases, injury prevention, and postexposure management.

Summary

Government regulations and recommendations have been developed with your best interests and health in mind. Today, the delivery of oral healthcare services requires that safety be an integral part of your daily routine.

In an effort to protect the health and safety of all employees, OSHA issued regulatory standards for healthcare facilities, including dental offices. These include hazardous chemical standards, industrial standards, and the Bloodborne Pathogens Standard. Other requirements affecting dental offices, such as waste disposal tracking, are governed by other federal, state, and local agencies.

HAZARDS

Exposure Control

If you're going to work in dentistry, you must accept the fact that you are going to be exposed to a variety of occupational hazards.

Can you think of one or two examples in your office in each of the four following areas?

Infectious Agents: _____

Chemicals: _____

Physical/Equipment: _____

Other: _____

To create a safe work environment, workplace hazards must be identified and managed to prevent exposure and potential injury. Exposure control reduces or eliminates the potential harm that may be encountered during the course of your job. The components of exposure control include:

Infection Control Policy and Practice   **Physical Precautions**

Chemical Safety   **Warning Signs or Labels**

Waste Management   **Record Keeping**

Each one of these component areas will be explained and/or demonstrated in detail during this course series. Exposure control is more than just infection control.

Infection Control: Infection control is a system of measures practiced by healthcare personnel, including dental health care personnel (DHCP) in healthcare facilities. The goals of infection control are to decrease transmission of infectious agents (e.g. bacteria, viruses, etc. that can produce infection). Infection control strategies are designed to prevent healthcare-associated infections in patients and injuries and illnesses in healthcare personnel. Infection control measures are based on how an infectious agent is transmitted and include standard, contact, droplet, and airborne precautions. Examples of infection control measures include proper hand hygiene, safe work practices, use of personal protective equipment (PPE) [masks or respirators, gloves, gowns, and eye protection]. CDC uses the terms *infection control* or *infection prevention* and *infection prevention and control* in its guidelines and other documents.

Exposure Control: Exposure control uses the concepts and strategies of infection control to prevent exposure to infectious agents and to limit the spread of infectious agents when exposure occurs. Exposure controls include administrative policies and procedures for infection control and safety, education and training, safe work practices, engineering controls, etc. OSHA uses the term *exposure control* throughout the Bloodborne Pathogens Standard. Dental settings are required to have a written exposure control plan and all employees must be familiar with its content.

A comprehensive infection prevention and safety program integrates infection control recommendations from the CDC infection control guidelines, and exposure control regulations from OSHA as well as other relevant standards and regulations at the state and local level.

Program Evaluation

Strategies and tools to evaluate your infection control and exposure control programs can include periodic observational assessments, checklists and routine review of occupational exposures to bloodborne pathogens. Evaluation offers opportunities to improve the effectiveness of your programs.

The Need For Training

It is only through training that a healthcare worker learns to protect himself or herself from on-the-job injuries and hazards. It is not only the responsibility of your employer to provide training, but it is also your obligation to learn the regulations and proper procedures.

Initial Training

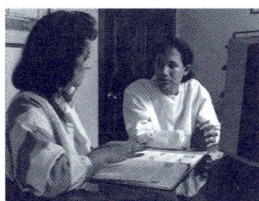

Initial training for any employee who may be exposed to infectious hazards or to hazardous chemicals must occur prior to performing any task involving these substances. OSHA requires employers to provide training at the time of initial assignment to tasks where occupational exposure may occur. Training must include discussions of the hazards associated with blood and other potentially infectious materials, chemical hazards, physical hazards, and waste management. This course forms the core of your initial training, and serves as reference material for detailed explanations and examples that are specific to your office.

Whenever there is a change in responsibilities, a change in office procedures where occupational hazards occur, or changes in government regulations, additional training must be provided specific to those changes.

Q&A

Question: *"I just started working here last week, after working at another dental practice. Can I continue to work without any training?"*

Answer: The experience you may have brought with you from another practice is valuable, and you can begin working with patients your first day on the job. However, you must be familiar with your new practice's infection control procedures, any chemicals used, and the location of critical equipment. It is required that all employees be fully trained to work in their new office environment prior to initial assignment to tasks where there is potential risk of exposure.

Annual Training

Training must occur at least once each year, facilitated by the employer or Infection Control Coordinator, to update employees on new information, technologies, equipment, and procedures. Annual training should also include materials not previously covered. In each training session, there should be opportunity for questions and answers and ample time for discussion. All training must be provided at no cost to the employee and during regular working hours by qualified individuals, in the appropriate language, with accurate, up-to-date materials.

3 Types of Training

Initial Training
- Whenever there is a change in responsibilities of staff or infection control coordinator
- Whenever there is a change in office procedures where there is a potential for an occupational exposure/hazard
- In response to changes in government regulations or recommendations

Additional Training
- When there are changes in policies, procedures, or products
- If new information is available or if there are changes in recommendations or regulations
- If someone does not follow standard operating procedures

Annual Training
- Required for specific OSHA standards such as the Bloodborne Pathogens Standard
- Recommended as good office policy

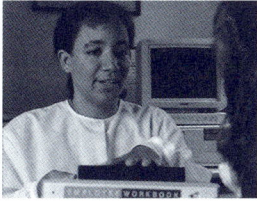

Your office has recently purchased a new environmental surface disinfectant. Before it can be used, each employee must receive product training which, at a minimum, must answer the following questions:

- *What are the brand and generic names of the product?*
- *Where is this product located?*
- *What are its major ingredients?*
- *When should this product be used?*
- *What are the procedures for its proper safe use?*
- *Are there any potential hazards?*
- *How can potential hazards be reduced?*
- *Where is the Safety Data Sheet (SDS) located?*
- *What are the first aid procedures for accidental exposure?*

Training Specific to Your Practice

This program, with its various integrated elements, provides a comprehensive training system to allow you and other employees to work in a safe and compliant manner. Part of this integration requires that your exposure control program be specific to your office, and include training and safety procedures that consider the uniqueness of your facility, local ordinances, special staff needs, and other constraints.

It is this program's intent to provide everyone in your practice new information and, at the same time, ensure that all office personnel possess, at a minimum, the knowledge base necessary to discuss safety and safe standard operating procedures. This program will also lead you step-by-step as your office customizes the material for governmental compliance. By following the guidelines set forth in this program, your office will be able to integrate exposure control into its daily routine with the least disruption of its day-to-day operations.

Infection Control Coordinator

To ensure the health and safety of everyone in your practice, an Infection Control Coordinator has been assigned to manage your practice's training program and to ensure that documentation is properly maintained. For training purposes, the Infection Control Coordinator is responsible for:

1 · **Scheduling and monitoring training for all personnel**
2 · **Maintaining training materials and records**
3 · **Customizing the course materials for the office setting**
4 · **Answering questions, and providing ongoing training**
The Infection Control Coordinator also communicates directly with OSAP if necessary.

Your office's Infection Control Coordinator is:

_____

The Infection Control/Exposure Control Plan is the core of your practice's training and safety program. Government regulations stipulate that all employees be aware of its content and prescribed procedures. Site specific infection control and safety program should integrate the OSHA Bloodborne Pathogens Standard and CDC recommendations. As you work through this training program, you and your Infection Control Coordinator will become familiar with all applicable regulations, either by creating a new Infection Control/Exposure Control Plan step- by-step or by adding to your office's existing plan. Your Infection Control/ Exposure Control Plan may contain:

- **Exposure Control Plan**
- **Exposure Determination**
- **Methods of Compliance**
- **Schedule of Implementation**
- **Documentation of Evaluation of Safety Devices**
- **Hazard Communication**
- **Emergency Procedures**
- **Waste Management Procedures**

The Infection Control/Exposure Control Plan for this practice is located:

_____

It is your Infection Control Coordinator's responsibility to ensure that your practice's written Infection Control/Exposure Control Plan reflects all policies and procedures. The success of the practice's safety program requires the cooperation of all staff members. As an ongoing role, the Coordinator will: supervise, evaluate and update the Plan as necessary; retrain all staff appropriately and supervise the training of new staff as they join the practice.

Need More Information?

This course series is written to give all employees, regardless of their experience, the same knowledge base in Exposure Control. Each course begins by outlining basic concepts and facts for the inexperienced healthcare worker, then logically builds on this material to the point where even experienced providers are learning new information.

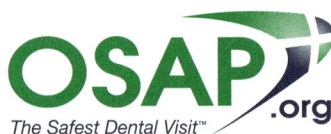

OSAP.org
The Safest Dental Visit™

For more information, visit the OSAP website at:
OSAP.org

In order to access the full resources of OSAP, you must maintain a current membership. Member benefits include publications (weekly "InfoBites", monthly infection control news summaries and bi-monthly *Infection Control in Practice TEAM HUDDLE™*); a password for the "Members-Only" section of the website with 60+ toolkits, charts and checklists, infection control practice tips, slide decks and videos; discounts on training materials and courses; complimentary access to "Ask OSAP" technical services and much more.

For more information about membership, visit the website at OSAP.org or call OSAP at 1-410-571-0003.

Discussion

Below are some questions that will assist you in a discussion with your Infection Control Coordinator or Safety Officer.

You have now completed the workbook segment for Course #1. Below are some questions that will also assist you in your discussion with your Infection Control Coordinator or dentist, and other staff members.

Question: *Will someone tell me when a patient has an infectious disease such as hepatitis, HIV, or influenza?*

Answer: You will not always know when or if a patient has an infectious disease such as hepatitis B, hepatitis C, HIV disease, tuberculosis or even influenza (the flu). There may be instances in which patients do not know they are infected, because symptoms may not yet have occurred. You should treat all patients as if they are infectious, and you should use precautions consistent with the recommended universal and standard precautions protocols.
(Standard Precautions: Course #2)

Question: *What are the different exposure control plans I need to know about?*

Answer: The primary types of exposure in a dental office are bloodborne/infectious/ biologic or chemical. OSHA has Standards which regulate both of these. One is the Bloodborne Pathogen Standards and the other is the Hazard Communication Standard. Each Standard requires an exposure control plan specific to each. The Hazard Communications Standard requires a written Hazard Communications Program and the Bloodborne Pathogens Standard requires a written Exposure Control Plan.

Question: *Infection Prevention, Infection Control, and Exposure Control – what are the differences?*

Answer: CDC, the federal agency that develops guidelines and recommendations to prevent and control infections and injuries, uses the terms *infection prevention, infection control* and uses *infection prevention and control*.
Infection prevention is designed to prevent healthcare-associated infections in patients and healthcare personnel through a variety of exposure prevention measures. Examples of prevention measures include a written infection prevention and control program, education, and training of personnel, immunizations,

personal protective equipment, safe work practices and use of devices with engineered safety features, sterility assurance of reusable patient care items, environmental cleaning and disinfection or use of surface barriers.

Infection control involves taking actions to reduce the risks associated with exposure to potentially infectious body fluids and materials. Examples of infection control measures include post-exposure management and medical follow-up. Although the concepts differ, the terms are often used interchangeably.

OSHA uses the term *Exposure Control*. OSHA requires employers to provide a place of employment either free of known hazards or when the hazards cannot be removed, protection from exposure to the hazards. Additionally OSHA regulates employers to manage exposures if they do occur and to reduce or limit the risks associated with the exposure. Exposure Control, as described by OSHA in the Bloodborne Pathogens Standard, consists of a variety of exposure prevention and management measures using the concept of universal precautions to reduce the employee's (e.g., healthcare worker's) risk of exposure to blood and other potentially infectious materials. These measures include education and training, hepatitis B vaccine, handwashing, personal protective equipment, use of engineering controls and work practice controls, etc.).

Each specific measure of infection prevention and control/exposure control is covered in detail in the following courses.

Objectives

Upon completion of this course on Occupational Exposure, you will be able to:

1. Explain three types of potential hazards in the oral healthcare setting.
2. Describe five primary types of control or protection methods to reduce on-the-job occupational exposure.
3. Identify the immunizations recommended by CDC for healthcare personnel.
4. Identify which CDC-recommended immunization(s) is/are regulated by OSHA.
5. Define standard precautions.
6. Differentiate standard precautions and universal precautions.
7. Define and provide two examples for each of the following terms:
   - Engineering Controls
   - Work Practice Controls
8. Identify two major bloodborne pathogens of concern.
9. Identify one major airborne pathogen of concern.
10. Identify three types of microorganisms associated with the transmission of disease.
11. Identify four factors affecting susceptibility to disease transmission.
12. Explain why different individuals may respond differently when exposed to the same type and dose of microorganism.
13. Identify two primary strategies of disease prevention.
14. Describe the requirements of the Needlestick Safety and Prevention act added to the Bloodborne Pathogens Standard in 2001 (i.e., assessing sharps safety devices).
15. Understand the process for screening and evaluating a new safety device.

Working in dentistry puts you at risk of potential exposure to a variety of hazards. These hazards may lead to an exposure incident with infectious materials, hazardous chemicals, and/or physical dangers, and could occur from various everyday activities from emptying the office trash to treating a patient who has an infectious disease.

Your day-to-day tasks may put you at risk of an *occupational exposure,* which can be divided into three basic areas: chemical, physical, and infectious. In addition, all three of these hazards may be present in dental waste. Each area carries with it a host of government regulations, recommendations, and professional standards. These require that you: 1) practice certain prescribed procedures in order to minimize risk, 2) be trained in these procedures by your employer, and 3) verify documentation of your office's policies, procedures, and training accomplishments. These three basic areas, together with waste management, form the core components of most health and safety issues affecting dental practices, and are the focus of this course series.

Hazards Targeted By Exposure Control

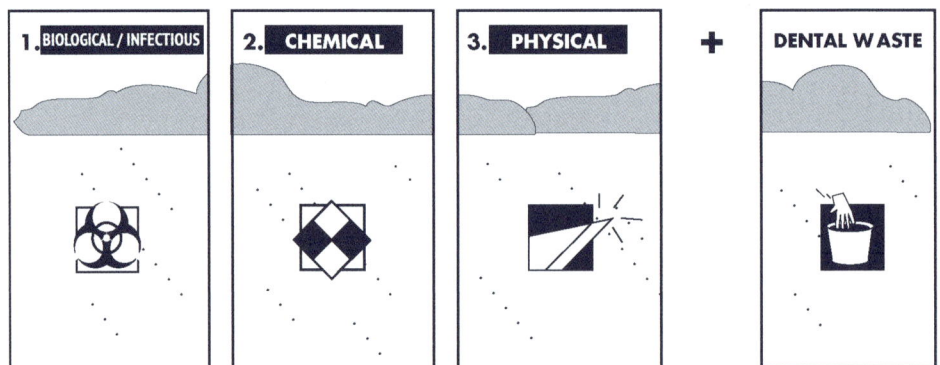

1. Biological / Infectious

Infectious diseases are a very real risk in the dental practice and must be taken seriously. The OSHA standard that impacts dental practices the greatest is the "Occupational Exposure to Bloodborne Pathogens Standard" 29 CFR Part 1910.1030. It is specific to *infectious disease exposure control* for preventing the transmission of bloodborne diseases. Previously, this was referred to as "Infection Control," but with the realization that the goal is to prevent exposure to infectious agents, the all-encompassing term is "Exposure Control." Exposure Control incorporates all the aspects of Infection Control with the related principles of occupational safety and health.

2. Chemical Hazards

Chemicals are used in every dental office; some are hazardous and others are not. The hazardous chemicals are regulated by OSHA in the "Hazard Communication Standard" CFR Part 1910.1200 (commonly called HAZCOM), by the federal Environmental Protection Agency (EPA), and by your state or local environmental agency. Your occupational exposure to chemicals in the dental office is limited by the use of *chemical exposure controls*: specific policies, procedures, and equipment designed to make your working environment as safe as possible.

The most visible portion of the regulations are the color-coded EPA/DOT (Dept. of Transportation) approved warning labels, however, these labels are just a part of the proper handling of chemicals in the workplace.

3. Physical Hazards

The design of your office and the equipment you use presents certain physical hazards. Are your electric wall outlets grounded? Is your evacuation system pump located the right distance from the system's filter? Are all your exits and non-exits clearly labeled? Do you have a fire escape plan? These and many other examples represent physical hazards that are governed by federal and state regulations, as well as local ordinances. OSHA is the primary agency involved in reducing the risk of physical injury. Other national codes such as those enacted by Building Officials & Code Administrators (BOCA), governing architects, and the National Fire Protection Association (NFPA), as well as governing fire codes, and additional state and local building codes, may also apply.

Another physical hazard, although remote, can occur with the use of X-ray devices, which creates a potential for exposure to ionizing radiation during the film exposure process. The use of radiation detection devices (film badges), appropriate standard operating procedures (SOPs), safe and properly maintained equipment, lead-lined walls, lead aprons, etc., are all used to prevent and protect you against exposure to ionizing radiation. In addition to the hazards associated with the exposing and processing of X-rays, there are also infectious hazards from potentially infectious saliva and contaminated exposed X-ray packages.

If your practice uses lasers, use standard precautions and follow manufacturers' directions for infection control and the prevention of exposure to infectious materials.

Hazard Example - Dental Waste

All three hazards described above can be found in dental waste. The waste you generate in your office may be chemical, biological, physical, or combinations of any of these. It is important to keep in mind that not all of the waste is hazardous or regulated. Most dental waste is considered general waste that is not likely to be infectious or hazardous.

Proper waste management is an integral part of your exposure control program. OSHA is primarily concerned with the manner in which you handle waste in order to reduce your risk of an exposure. Other federal, state, and local authorities govern the packaging requirements, transportation, and disposal of dental waste. Once you understand the type of waste you are dealing with, you can implement the proper disposal and tracking requirements. Dental waste is covered in course #7.

What are the three areas of Occupational Exposure that are of concern in your dental practice?

1. _____

2. _____

3. _____

Each of the three areas above has specific regulatory requirements that mandate special procedures within your dental office. In the process of learning and then practicing safe and practical office procedures, you should meet the requirements of all applicable regulations.

Controls

The primary purpose of employee health and safety policies, procedures and regulations is to reduce the probability of occupational exposure to blood, potentially infectious materials, hazardous chemicals, and physical hazards. The process of reducing on-the-job risks (occupational exposure) is called either Exposure Control (Bloodborne Pathogens Standard) or Hazard Abatement (Hazard Communication Standard). The five primary controls or protection methods for this are:

1) **Universal/Standard Precautions**
2) **Work Practice Controls**
3) **Engineering Controls**
4) **Personal Protective Equipment**
5) **Environmental Infection Control**
 · **Clinical Contact Surfaces**
 · **Housekeeping Surfaces**

Universal Precautions/Standard Precautions

Universal Precautions are a method of infection control based on the concept that all blood and body fluids that might be contaminated with blood should be treated as infectious. These precautions apply to bloodborne hazards that may be associated with a percutaneous exposure (needlestick), a splash to the eyes, nose or mouth; or contact with nonintact skin.

OSHA uses the term *Universal Precautions* but CDC now uses the term *Standard Precautions*.

Standard Precautions are similar to Universal Precautions in that they apply to all patients, blood, and bloodborne body fluids. Standard Precautions use and expand the elements of Universal Precautions into a standard of care to protect both healthcare workers and patients. Standard Precautions are infection prevention practices based on the principle that all blood, body fluids, secretions, excretions (except sweat), non-intact skin, and mucous membranes may be infectious. These precautions are applied when treating all patients, whether they appear sick or healthy. Standard precautions include hand hygiene; use of personal protective equipment; respiratory hygiene and cough etiquette; safe injection practices; and the safe handling of potentially contaminated equipment or surfaces in the patient environment.

Saliva has always been considered a potentially infectious material in dental infection control; thus, no operational difference exists in clinical dental practice between universal precautions and standard precautions.

Universal/Standard Precautions assume that all patients and all materials are potentially infectious. Because of this, you must make every effort to protect yourself at all times. Universal/Standard Precautions are the cornerstone of infection control and serve as your most important protection concept. These precautions must be part of other control methods such as work practice controls and engineering controls.

Work Practice Controls

The way you handle needles, wash your hands or carry contaminated instruments can either be done in a safe or unsafe manner. *Work Practice Controls* (also called safe work practices) are safe work habits; those methods of performing a task that reduce the chance of an exposure incident. Each office should develop practice-specific standardized procedures that protect employees and patients from accidents, physical injuries, and exposure to chemical and infectious hazards. Safe and accepted Work Practice Controls are covered more specifically in Course #4.

Engineering Controls

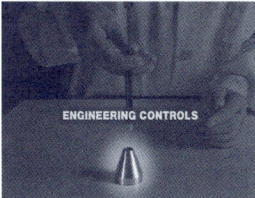

Work Practice Controls may not always ensure a completely safe working environment. Safe work habits should be combined with the use of equipment and devices that isolate or prevent an injury. An *Engineering Control* is a device, piece of equipment, or technology that removes or isolates a hazard in the workplace. It is critical that you be initially trained and then retrained annually in the proper use of dental equipment. Engineering Controls must be examined and maintained or replaced on a regular schedule to ensure effectiveness. Engineering Controls are covered throughout this course series. Equipment considerations, limitations, and selection are covered in Course #6.

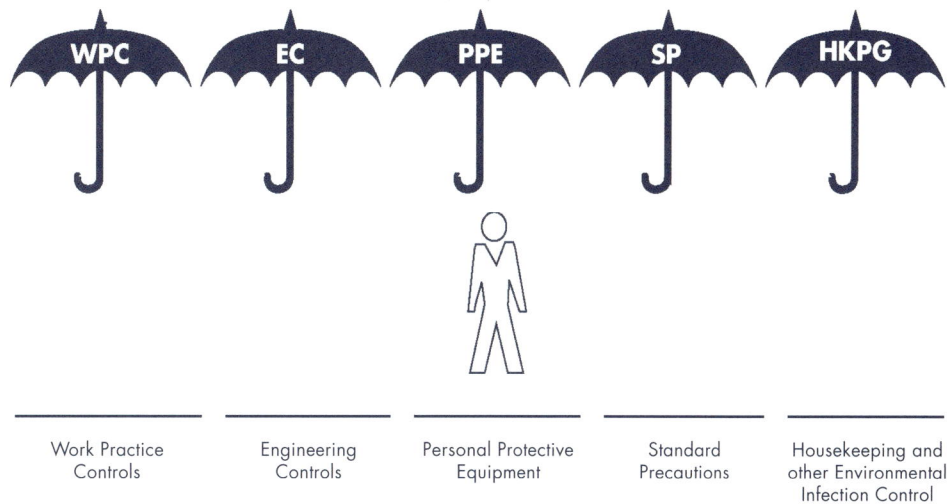

WPC	EC	PPE	SP	HKPG
Work Practice Controls	Engineering Controls	Personal Protective Equipment	Standard Precautions	Housekeeping and other Environmental Infection Control

Personal Protective Equipment

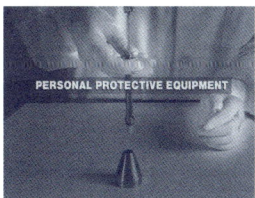

There is a wide variety of appropriate Personal Protective Equipment (PPE) to protect yourself against the risk of occupational exposure. These include gloves, masks, eyewear, and clinical clothing. PPE is covered in detail in Course #3.

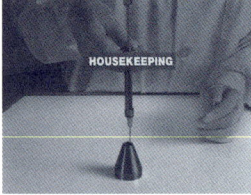

OSHA's Bloodborne Pathogens Standard states: "Employers shall ensure that the worksite is maintained in a clean and sanitary condition." Environmental surfaces are either Clinical Contact or Housekeeping. These tasks include cleaning clinical area and the handling of regulated waste and laundry. Each of these areas are covered in later courses and have corresponding written procedures in the Update text to read: Infection Control/Exposure Control Plan. Environmental Infection Control is covered in greater depth in course #4.

Example:

Allison has recently been hired as a new dental assistant, and one of her designated tasks is instrument recirculation (also called instrument reprocessing). She uses the heat sterilizer (an Engineering Control) and must be trained to properly handle contaminated instruments and operate the heat sterilizer (Work Practice Controls). The worksite should be clear of unnecessary items and cleaned regularly (Housekeeping). Allison wears heavy duty utility gloves, protective eyewear, and clothing appropriate for each step of the sterilization process: carrying and cleaning instruments, operating the sterilizer and removing instruments from the sterilizer (PPE).

In most cases, physical and chemical hazards are relatively easy to identify when compared to the unseen hazards associated with infectious agents and contaminated materials. While all three risks will be covered in greater detail in other courses in this workbook the remainder of this course deals specifically with risks associated with bloodborne infectious agents and how to control them.

What is the storage location of each of the following pieces of PPE in your work space?

Gloves: _____

Masks: _____

Clothing: _____

Eyewear: _____

Other: _____

Process of Disease Transmission

How diseases are transmitted from one person to another determines the procedures used for infection control in dentistry. Microorganisms such as bacteria, viruses and fungi are found throughout the body and can be carried by blood, saliva, or other body fluids. In the dental setting, exposure incidents may result from contact with blood, body fluids, or other potentially infectious materials that can occur through direct contact, indirect contact, and/or spatter and aerosols. OSHA defines an "occupational exposure" incident as:

"A specific eye, mouth, mucous membrane, nonintact skin, or parenteral (puncture wounds) contact with blood or other potentially infectious materials that results from the performance of an employee's duties." (29 CFR 1910.1030 Pg. 64175; "Bloodborne Pathogens, Final Rule" of December 6, 1991)

Hosts and Agents

The ability of an organism to infect and cause disease depends on both the potential host and the infectious agent. A host is a potentially infected person and an agent is a microorganism. After being exposed to an agent, a host (you, for example) may be infected, but may not develop actual disease. The biggest factors affecting your resistance to disease are your general health and status of your immune system, and depending on your resistance, you may or may not develop actual disease.

The ability of an agent to infect you is a function of the type of microorganism and its virulence (its ability to overcome body defenses), as well as the actual amount transmitted (dosage). Fortunately, most infections, whether bacterial, viral, or fungal, are handled effectively by the body's own defense mechanisms.

HOST ——————————— **AGENTS**

Resistance depends on:
· General Health
· Status of Immune System

Ability to infect depends on:
· Dosage (Amount)
· Virulence (Strength)

Transmission

The route of disease transmission in dentistry is more likely to be via blood or other body fluids, air, or water. *Transmission* occurs when an organism enters the body through various routes, for example: contact with chapped skin (direct contact), splashes to the eye or nose (mucous membrane), inhalation to the throat or lung (aerosol contact), ingestion of food or water, skin wound, needlestick (parenteral contact), or other means.

After transmission, most bacteria are easily defeated by the body's (or the new host's) defense mechanisms or by use of antibiotics, antiviral or anti-fungal agents taken after infection occurs. *Viruses*, the smallest of all microorganisms, are not as easily defeated, and cause diseases such as measles, smallpox, polio, viral hepatitis, rabies, herpes, flu/influenza, and HIV disease.

Each virus contains a central core of nucleic acid (DNA or RNA) and an outer cover of protein. It is this inner nucleic acid core that actually causes infection. While viruses are completely dependent on animal, plant, or bacterial host cells for survival and reproduction, once established, these viruses can actually reattach themselves to new, healthy host cells, and then penetrate and infect them.

Your immune status is a major factor in determining your risk of infection after an exposure to blood containing an infectious microorganism. Without immunization, your risk of infection depends upon the risk associated with the particular microorganism. If you are immunized, the balance is tipped in your favor.

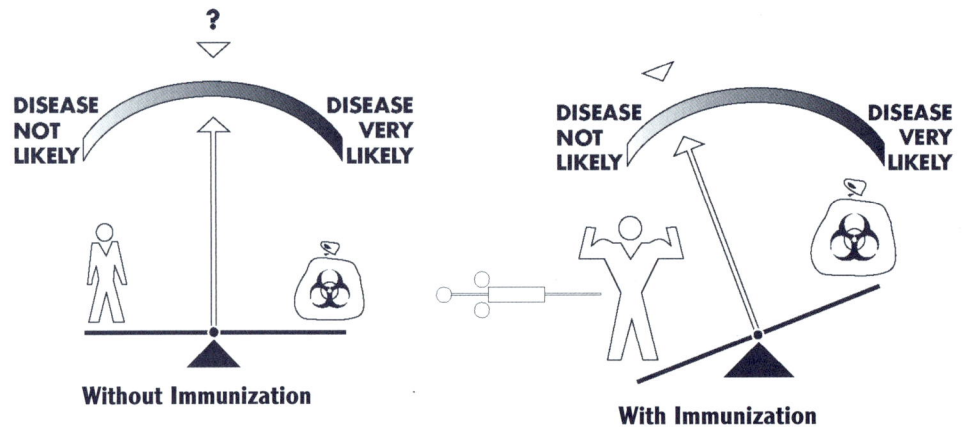

Without Immunization   **With Immunization**

Protecting Yourself

To defeat a virus, the body's internal defense mechanisms must either inactivate all of the agent's cells on its own (antiviral agents are in some cases useful against certain viruses) or be immune to the virus through previous infection or immunization (if available for that specific disease). See CDC Recommended Immunizations on next page.

The best of all options, however, is to prevent the infection in the first place through Exposure Control, which includes the Hazard Abatement components of Universal/Standard Precautions, Work Practice Controls, Engineering Controls, PPE, and Housekeeping (Environmental Infection Control).

Sepsis is the body's extreme response to an infection. It is a life-threatening medical emergency. Sepsis happens when an infection you already have–in your skin, lungs, urinary tract, or somewhere else–triggers a chain reaction throughout your body. Without timely treatment, sepsis can rapidly lead to tissue damage, organ failure, and death. The following links provide the most current information on sepsis.

Source: Accessed July 2019

Asepsis and Prevention

https://www.cdc.gov/sepsis/index.html

https://www.sepsis.org/sepsis-and/dental-health

Bloodborne Disease Transmission

The bloodborne pathogens of primary concern to healthcare workers are hepatitis B virus (HBV), hepatitis C virus (HCV), and human immunodeficiency virus (HIV). To date, the only available vaccine for a bloodborne pathogen is the hepatitis B vaccine. There are also a number of other vaccine-preventable diseases against which you should be protected. Please see Table 2 in this course for the CDC-recommended immunizations for healthcare personnel.

CDC Recommended Immunizations for Health-Care Personnel (HCP)

MMWR / November 25, 2011 / Vol. 60 / No. 7
http://www.cdc.gov/mmwr/preview/mmwrhtml/rr6007a1.htm?s_cid=rr6007a1_e#Tab2

TABLE 2. Immunizing agents and immunization schedules for health-care personnel (HCP)*

Generic name	Primary schedule and booster(s)	Indications	Major precautions and contraindications	Special considerations
Immunizing agents recommended for all HCP				
Hepatitis B (HB) recombinant vaccine	2 doses 4 weeks apart; third dose 5 months after second; booster doses not necessary; all doses should be administered IM in the deltoid	Preexposure: HCP at risk for exposure to blood or body fluids; postexposure (see Table 4)	On the basis of limited data, no risk for adverse effects to developing fetuses is apparent. Pregnancy should not be considered a contraindication to vaccination of women. Previous anaphylactic reaction to common baker's yeast is a contraindication to vaccination.	The vaccine produces neither therapeutic nor adverse effects in HBV-infected persons. Prevaccination serologic screening is not indicated for persons being vaccinated because of occupational risk but might be indicated for HCP in certain high-risk populations. HCP at high risk for occupational† contact with blood or body fluids should be tested 1–2 months after vaccination to determine serologic response.
Hepatitis B immune globulin (HBIG)	0.06 mL/kg IM as soon as possible after exposure, if indicated	Postexposure prophylaxis (see Table 4)	See package insert§	
Influenza vaccine (TIV and LAIV)	Annual vaccination with current seasonal vaccine. TIV is available in IM and ID formulations. LAIV is administered intranasally.	All HCP	History of severe (e.g., anaphylactic) hypersensitivity to eggs; prior severe allergic reaction to influenza vaccine	No evidence exists of risk to mother of fetus when the vaccine is administered to a pregnant woman with an underlying high-risk condition. Influenza vaccination is recommended for women who are or will be pregnant during influenza season because of increased risk for hospitalization and death. LAIV is recommended only for healthy, non-pregnant persons aged 2–49 years. Intradermal vaccine is indicated for persons aged 18–64 years. HCP who care for severely immunosuppressed persons who require a protective environment should receive TIV rather than LAIV.
Measles live-virus vaccine	2 doses SC; ≥28 days apart	Vaccination should be recommended for all HCP who lack presumptive evidence of immunity;¶ vaccination should be considered for those born before 1957.	Pregnancy; immunocompromised persons,** including HIV-infected persons who have evidence of severe immunosuppression; anaphylaxis to gelatin or gelatin-containing products; anaphylaxis to neomycin; and recent administration of immune globulin.	HCP vaccinated during 1963–1967 with a killed measles vaccine alone, killed vaccine followed by live vaccine, or a vaccine of unknown type should be revaccinated with 2 doses of live measles virus vaccine.
Mumps live-virus vaccine	2 doses SC; ≥28 days apart	Vaccination should be recommended for all HCP who lack presumptive evidence of immunity.†† Vaccination should be considered for those born before 1957.	Pregnancy; immunocompromised persons,** including HIV-infected persons who have evidence of severe immunosuppression; anaphylaxis to gelatin or gelatin-containing products; anaphylaxis to neomycin	HCP vaccinated before 1979 with either killed mumps vaccine or mumps vaccine of unknown type should consider revaccination with 2 doses of MMR vaccine.
Rubella live-virus vaccine	1 dose SC; (However, due to the 2-dose requirements for measles and mumps vaccines, the use of MMR vaccine will result in most HCP receiving 2 doses of rubella-containing vaccine.)	Vaccination should be recommended for all HCP who lack presumptive evidence of immunity.§§	Pregnancy; immunocompromised persons** including HIV-infected persons who have evidence of severe immunosuppression; anaphylaxis to gelatin or gelatin-containing products; anaphylaxis to neomycin	The risk for rubella vaccine-associated malformations in the offspring of women pregnant when vaccinated or who become pregnant within 1 month after vaccination is negligible.¶¶ Such women should be counseled regarding the theoretical basis of concern for the fetus.
Tetanus and diphtheria (toxoids) and acellular pertussis (Tdap)	1 dose IM as soon as feasible if Tdap not already received and regardless of interval from last Td. After receipt of Tdap, receive Td for routine booster every 10 years.	All HCP, regardless of age.	History of serious allergic reaction (i.e., anaphylaxis) to any component of Tdap. Because of the importance of tetanus vaccination, persons with history of anaphylaxis to components in Tdap or Td should be referred to an allergist to determine whether they have a specific allergy to tetanus toxoid and can safely receive tetanus toxoid (TT) vaccine. Persons with history of encephalopathy (e.g., coma or prolonged seizures) not attributable to an identifiable cause within 7 days of administration of a vaccine with pertussis components should receive Td instead of Tdap.	Tetanus prophylaxis in wound management if not yet received Tdap***
Varicella vaccine (varicella zoster virus live-virus vaccine)	2 doses SC 4–8 weeks apart if aged ≥13 years.	All HCP who do not have evidence of immunity defined as: written documentation of vaccination with 2 doses of varicella vaccine; laboratory evidence of immunity††† or laboratory confirmation of disease; diagnosis or verification of a history of varicella disease by a health-care provider;§§§ or diagnosis or verification of a history of herpes zoster by a health-care provider.	Pregnancy; immunocompromised persons,** history of anaphylactic reaction after receipt of gelatin or neomycin. Varicella vaccination may be considered for HIV-infected adolescents and adults with CD4+ T-lymphocyte count >200 cells/uL. Avoid salicylate use for 6 weeks after vaccination.	Because 71%–93% of adults without a history of varicella are immune, serologic testing before vaccination is likely to be cost-effective.
Varicella-zoster immune globulin	125U/10 kg IM (minimum dose: 125U; maximum dose: 625U)	Persons without evidence of immunity who have contraindications for varicella vaccination and who are at risk for severe disease and complications¶¶¶ known or likely to be susceptible who have direct, nontransient exposure to an infectious hospital staff worker or patient		Serologic testing may help in assessing whether to administer varicella-zoster immune globulin. If use of varicella-zoster immune globulin prevents varicella disease, patient should be vaccinated subsequently. The varicella-zoster immune globulin product currently used in the United States (VariZIG) (Cangene Corp. Winnipeg Canada) can be obtained 24 hours a day from the sole authorized U.S. distributor (FFF Enterprises, Temecula, California) at 1-800-843-7477 or http://www.fffenterprises.com
Other immunobiologics that might be indicated in certain circumstances for HCP				
Quadrivalent meningococcal conjugate vaccine (tetravalent (A,C,Y,W) for HCP ages 19–54 years, Quadrivalent meningococcal polysaccharide vaccine for HCP age >55 years	1 dose; booster dose in 5 years if person remains at increased risk	Clinical and research microbiologists who might routinely be exposed to isolates of Neisseria meningitidis	The safety of the vaccine in pregnant women has not been evaluated; it should not be administered during pregnancy unless the risk for infection is high.	

TABLE 2. *(Continued)* Immunizing agents and immunization schedules for health-care personnel (HCP)*

Generic name	Primary schedule and booster(s)	Indications	Major precautions and contraindications	Special considerations
Typhoid vaccine IM, and oral	IM vaccine: 1 dose, booster every 2 years. Oral vaccine: 4 doses on alternate days. Manufacturer recommends revaccination with the entire 4-dose series every 5 years.	Workers in microbiology laboratories who frequently work with *Salmonella typhi*.	Severe local or systemic reaction to a previous dose. Ty21a (oral) vaccine should not be administered to immunocompromised persons** or to persons receiving antimicrobial agents.	Vaccination should not be considered an alternative to the use of proper procedures when handling specimens and cultures in the laboratory.
Inactivated poliovirus vaccine (IPV)	For unvaccinated adults, 2 doses should be administered at intervals of 4–8 weeks; a third dose should be administered 6–12 months after the second dose.	Vaccination is recommended for adults at increased risk for exposure to polioviruses including health-care personnel who have close contact with patients who might be excreting polioviruses. Adults who have previously received a complete course of poliovirus vaccine may receive one lifetime booster if they remain at increased risk for exposure.	Hypersensitivity or anaphylactic reactions to IPV or antibiotics contained in IPV. IPV contains trace amounts of streptomycin, polymyxin B, and neomycin.	

Abbreviations: IM = intramuscular; HBV = hepatitis B virus; HBsAg = hepatitis B surface antigen; SC = subcutaneous; HIV = human immunodeficiency virus; MMR = measles, mumps, rubella vaccine; TB = tuberculosis; HAV = hepatitis A virus; IgA = immune globulin A; ID = intradermal; TIV = trivalent inactivated split-virus vaccines; LAIV = live attenuated influenza vaccine; BCG = bacille Calmette-Guérin; OPV = oral poliovirus vaccine.
* Persons who provide health care to patients or work in institutions that provide patient care (e. g., physicians, nurses, emergency medical personnel, dental professionals and students, medical and nursing students, laboratory technicians, hospital volunteers, and administrative and support staff in health-care institutions). **Source:** U.S. Department of Health and Human Services. Definition of health-care personnel (HCP). Available at: http://www.hhs.gov/ash/initiatives/hai/hcpflu.html

† Health-care personnel and public safety workers at high risk for continued percutaneous or mucosal exposure to blood or body fluids include acupuncturists, dentists, dental hygienists, emergency medical technicians, first responders, laboratory technologists/technicians, nurses, nurse practitioners, phlebotomists, physicians, physician assistants, and students entering these professions. **Source:** CDC. A comprehensive immunization strategy to eliminate transmission of hepatitis B virus infection in the United States: recommendations of the Advisory Committee on Immunization Practices. Part II: immunization of adults. MMWR 2006;55(No. RR-16).

§ The package insert should be consulted to weigh the risks and benefits of giving HBIG to persons with IgA deficiency, or to persons who have had an anaphylactic reaction to an IgG containing biologic product.

¶ Written documentation of vaccination with 2 doses of live measles or MMR vaccine administered ≥28 days apart, or laboratory evidence of measles immunity, or laboratory confirmation of measles disease, or birth before 1957.

** Persons immunocompromised because of immune deficiency diseases, HIV infection (who should primarily not receive BCG, OPV, and yellow fever vaccines), leukemia, lymphoma or generalized malignancy or immunosuppressed as a result of therapy with corticosteroids, alkylating drugs, antimetabolites, or radiation.

†† Written documentation of vaccination with 2 doses of live mumps or MMR vaccine administered ≥28 days apart, or laboratory evidence of mumps immunity, or laboratory confirmation of mumps disease, or birth before 1957.

§§ Written documentation of vaccination with 1 dose of live rubella or MMR vaccine, or laboratory evidence of immunity, or laboratory confirmation of rubella infection or disease, or birth before 1957, except women of childbearing potential who could become pregnant; though pregnancy in this age group would be exceedingly rare.

¶¶ **Source:** CDC. Revised ACIP recommendation for avoiding pregnancy after receiving a rubella-containing vaccine. MMWR 2001;50:1117.

*** **Source:** CDC. Update on adult immunization: recommendations of the Advisory Committee on Immunization Practices (ACIP). MMWR 1991;40(No. RR-12).

††† Commercial assays can be used to assess disease-induced immunity, but they often lack sensitivity to detect vaccine-induced immunity (i.e., they might yield false-negative results).

§§§ Verification of history or diagnosis of typical disease can be provided by any health-care provider (e.g., school or occupational clinic nurse, nurse practitioner, physician assistant, or physician). For persons reporting a history of, or reporting with, atypical or n assessment by a physician or their designee is recommended, and one of the following should be sought: 1) an epidemiologic link to a typical varicella case or to a laboratory--confirmed case or 2) evidence of laboratory confirmation if it was performed at the tim disease. When such documentation is lacking, persons should not be considered as having a valid history of disease because other diseases might mimic mild atypical varicella.

¶¶¶ For example, immunocompromised patients or pregnant women.

For more information on the recommended adolescent and adult immunization schedule go to www.cdc.gov/vaccines/hcp/acip-recs/index.html

Special Note: MMR (Measles, Mumps, & Rubella)

If you were born in 1957 or later and have not had the MMR vaccine, or if you don't have an up-to-date blood test that shows you are immune to measles or mumps (i.e., no serologic evidence of immunity or prior vaccination), get 2 doses of MMR (1 dose now and the 2nd dose at least 28 days later).

If you were born in 1957 or later and have not had the MMR vaccine, or if you don't have an up-to-date blood test that shows you are immune to rubella, only 1 dose of MMR is recommended. However, you may end up receiving 2 doses, because the rubella component is in the combination vaccine with measles and mumps. For HCWs born before 1957, see the MMR ACIP vaccine recommendations

People who previously had one or two doses of MMR vaccine can still get mumps and transmit the disease.

Source: www.cdc.gov/mumps/hcp.html

Cross Contamination/Cross Infection:

Cross-infection or contamination occurs when you, or your patient, has an infection and that infection is passed along to other staff members, family, friends or other patients.

Cross-infection can occur in dental settings when infection control practices are not followed or when sterilization failures occur. Infected material left behind on clinical surfaces, unsterilized instruments, or other items can be transmitted to staff and other patients. Several highly-publicized cases of cross-infection between patients, sometimes called patient-to-patient transmission, have occurred in healthcare settings and have been linked to lapses in infection control.

Hepatitis

Hepatitis is inflammation of the liver caused by viruses, bacteria, toxins, certain drugs, autoimmune diseases or physical injury. Although many hepatitis patients have no signs or symptoms of the disease, some develop jaundice, a yellowing of the skin, mucous membranes and the eyes. Hepatitis can result in fibrosis and scarring of the liver (cirrhosis) and cancer. Currently, hepatitis caused by the hepatitis B virus (HBV) or the hepatitis C virus (HCV) are of greatest infection prevention and control concern in dental settings.

Hepatitis B Background

The hepatitis B virus (HBV) is highly infectious and is the most common occupational disease acquired in a dental setting. CDC estimated about 20,900 new infections of HBV occurred in 2016 and about 1.2 million people had chronic HBV infection. As many as 50% of these individuals are not even aware that they are infected. Approximately 25% of persons with chronic HBV infection die prematurely from cirrhosis or liver cancer.

HBV infection is a serious public health issue. The good news is that acute HBV infections declined over 80% since 1991 when the US began a national effort to fight HBV infection and began routine vaccination of children. However, dental health care personnel (DHCP) must still be aware of the risk of transmission while treating patients.

Hepatitis B Transmission

DHCP have almost daily contact with instruments and dental operatory waste that may be contaminated with hepatitis B. Unprotected DHCP who have not been vaccinated against HBV or do not respond to the vaccine are at a higher risk of becoming infected.

HBV is highly infectious and can continue to be infectious outside the body for at least 7 days. HBV infection can be spread through skin punctures from needlesticks or intravenous drug use, through direct contact with mucous membranes or when nonintact skin (e.g., psoriasis, eczema, burns, wounds, cuts, and scratches) is exposed to infectious blood or body fluids, even when there is no visible blood. HBV infection, however, does not spread through water, food, sharing eating utensils, sneezing or coughing.

The risk of HBV infection from a needlestick ranges from 60 to 300 transmissions out of 1000 needlesticks. Although HBV is highly infectious, CDC reports that from 1983 to 2010, the number of HBV infections among healthcare workers declined about 98%. This is a result of increases in healthcare worker immunization and may also be associated with compliance with infection control recommendations.

Note:

Hepatitis D virus (HDV), also referred to as Delta Hepatitis, can only occur in someone infected with hepatitis B. It is a defective virus that depends on hepatitis B for transmission. However, co-infection of hepatitis D often results in a more serious and potentially more often fatal course of disease. Protection against hepatitis B by immunization also protects against hepatitis D infection.

Although this disease has not reached epidemic proportions in the US, hepatitis B is an epidemic in many areas of the world. Because we live in a transient society, there is a potential risk of being in contact with hepatitis B on a daily basis, either knowingly or unknowingly. It is comforting to know that you can avoid this disease through the simple steps of being immunized and following safe office procedures. Immunizations are extremely effective against hepatitis B, and the OSHA Bloodborne Pathogens Standard of 1991 stipulates that all healthcare employers must make available and pay for hepatitis B immunizations for all employees who have the potential to be exposed (as recommended by the United States Public Health Service [USPHS]).

HAZARDS

HBV IMMUNIZED   NOT HBV IMMUNIZED

You have the right to refuse this immunization, however, to underscore the seriousness of this simple preventive measure and to meet government regulations, your refusal must be in writing on an OSHA-designated Hepatitis B Vaccination Declination Waiver Form, to be found in your office's Infection Control/Exposure Control Plan. The immunization may only be refused after the employee is informed of the safety and efficacy of the vaccine and the potential risk of refusing vaccination. If you do refuse the immunization and sign the form, you still have the right, at any time, to change your mind and receive the immunization series, at your employer's expense.

The Immunization Process is Simple and Straightforward:

1 · A blood test may be taken before immunization to determine your immunity status to HBV (titer). While this pre-immunization titer is not routinely recommended by CDC for those being immunized for occupational risk, your physician may decide to recommend this test.

2 · You will receive three injections; all of these shots should be given intramuscularly in your arm and at your employer's expense:
   · Initial dose (day 1)
   · Second dose one month later (day 30)
   · Third dose six months after the first dose (day 180)

3 · CDC recommends an HBV post-immunization antibody titer test for healthcare personnel who may have blood, patient or sharp instrument contact. This can be done one to two months after the last injection of HBV vaccine to determine your immune response and adequate antibody levels. Until the final results of this HBV surface antibody test are complete, you should assume that you are not immune. CDC also recommends that any healthcare personnel who were previously immunize , but did

not have a post-immunization antibody titer, have an antibody titer test. If the titer indicates inadequate antibody levels, an additional dose of vaccine or the entire series should be provided, followed by another HBV antibody titer test. OSHA regulates that the immunization series and antibody titer test be provided by the employer at no cost to the employee.

4 · The CDC does not currently recommend booster doses for persons with normal immune status who have been vaccinated.

Note:

For approximately 4-6% of individuals, the HBV immunization will not "take." An attending physician may recommend a second 3-dose vaccine series, however approximately 66% of the 4-6% will not develop the immunity. These persons are called non-responders as they do not develop immunity against hepatitis B, and are only protected through proper use of barrier techniques and other methods of infection control. If you appear to be a non-responder, you may wish to consult an infectious disease specialist. Individuals may not respond to the vaccine because they are already infected with the HBV (i.e., are chronic carriers).

Hepatitis C Transmission

In the 1970s, hepatitis viruses that could not be identified as either HAV or HBV were referred to as non-A non-B hepatitis (NANBH). In 1989, hepatitis C was isolated and identified as one of the major NANBH viruses. Hepatitis C is spread primarily through blood contact and to a lesser extent through sexual transmission or during pregnancy. The risk of transmission after a needlestick is lower than the risk associated with HBV exposure.

Healthcare workers are not at an increased occupational risk for hepatitis C. The level of infection among healthcare workers is similar to or lower than that of the general public. There is no vaccine or postexposure treatment available, as is available for hepatitis B. However, there are new antiretroviral agents to treat HCV in an infected person. Prevention requires the establishment of policies and procedures, including training and following proper exposure control recommendations with regard to preventing bloodborne disease transmission.

HIV

Human immunodeficiency virus (HIV), the virus associated with Acquired Immune Deficiency Syndrome (AIDS), is transmitted via body fluids in a manner similar to hepatitis B. Signs and symptoms of early HIV infection such as malaise, fever, night sweats, diarrhea and others may mimic the flu or other infections. CDC estimates that about 13% of persons with HIV are unaware of their status and recommends routine testing of all individuals from age 13-65 regardless of risk. Rapid HIV tests are available that can provide results in about 20 minutes.

The risk of HIV transmission in the dental setting is very low. CDC reports that the risk of HIV transmission from splashes with body fluids is about zero, even if the fluids are bloody. For healthcare personnel, less than 3 out of 1000 needle-stick injuries result in HIV infection. In comparison, the risks for hepatitis among nonimmunized healthcare personnel are higher, ranging from 60 to 300 transmissions out of 1000 needlesticks.

Potential Transmission Risks to Healthcare Workers

Pathogen	Concentration/ml in Serum Plasma	Transmission Rate (%) After Needlestick Injury
HBV	1,000,000 - 100,000,000	6.0 - 31.0
HCV	10 - 1,000,000	1.8
HIV	10 - 1,000	0.3

HIV Preventive Measures

Currently, there is no immunization against HIV. Although occupational transmission of HIV to healthcare workers is extremely rare, you must rely on strict compliance with safe procedures to protect yourself, other staff and your patients.

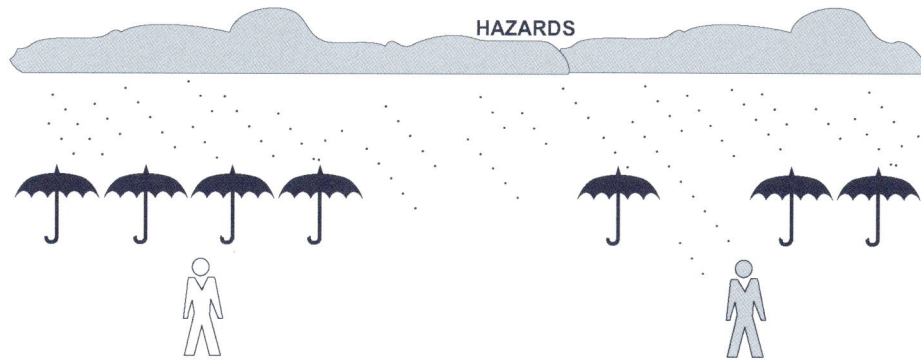

HAZARDS

The use of PPE and safety devices designed to prevent injuries from sharp medical devices can help minimize the risk of exposure. For workers who are exposed, CDC has developed recommendations to minimize the risk of developing HIV.

Other HIV Concerns

HIV infection has significant importance for dentistry because there are many different ways that the infection will show symptoms in the mouth. In fact, the DCHP may be the first person to suspect or recognize associated symptoms of HIV infection or failure of HIV treatment, which may allow the patient to receive an early diagnosis and seek medical treatment.

Multi-drug regimens now available for persons with HIV have significantly impacted their health and have reduced the progression to AIDS. In other words, persons with HIV are staying healthier. These same drugs have been recommended for use in postexposure management, which is discussed later in this chapter.

Other than for direct patient care or discussion within the office, a person's known or suspected HIV status should not be disclosed without written informed consent. In most states, this is a matter of law and there is no exception, even for purposes of evaluating an occupational exposure.

Airborne Disease Transmission

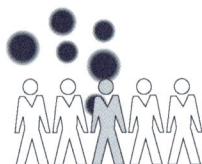

In 1994 the CDC released guidelines for preventing transmission of *Mycobacterium tuberculosis* (TB) in healthcare facilities, including dental facilities. As a result of compliance with this guideline, there has been a decrease in healthcare-associated transmission of TB. The TB guidelines were updated in 2005 to broaden the scope of healthcare facilities and discuss changes in testing, screening, explanation of new terms (airborne precautions), to provide information on multidrug resistant TB (MDR TB) and HIV infection and to review training and education. Dental staff are among those CDC lists as being part of a TB screening program. These guidelines emphasize the need for a TB infection control program and discuss the recommended control measures.

Your office's specific TB infection control program depends on the risk associated with TB in your community or in your facility. Information on your community is available through your state or local health department. Information on your facility would include a review of the number, if any, active TB patients encountered in your practice within at least the five previous years. Results of this assessment will determine your risk for TB transmission and help design your control program. In general, most dental facilities, unless they treat persons with active TB, are considered low risk.

Transmission and Pathogenesis

Tuberculosis is a clinical illness caused by the bacterium *M. tuberculosis*. Effective prevention and control of *M. tuberculosis* is based on a clear understanding of how TB is transmitted, how infection becomes established, and how infection progresses to clinical disease. *M. tuberculosis* is spread through airborne particles, known as droplet nuclei, that can be generated when persons with pulmonary or laryngeal TB sneeze, cough, speak, or sing. The particles are extremely small in size, and normal air currents can keep them airborne for prolonged time periods, spreading them throughout a room or building. Infection may occur when a person inhales droplet nuclei containing TB bacilli, which may reach the alveoli, where infection begins. Within two to ten weeks, the body's immunologic response to TB bacilli usually prevents further multiplication and spreading. This condition is referred to as *latent TB infection*.

Persons with *latent TB infection* usually have a positive skin test to tuberculin purified protein derivative (PPD), do not have active TB, and cannot infect others. In the U.S., about 90% of infected persons remain infected for life, with no progression to active TB. In about 5% of recently infected persons, active TB disease will develop in the first year or two after infection, and another 5% will develop disease later in life. The risk of developing active TB varies with age and immunologic status. In 2019 CDC updated the recommendations for ongoing or annual testing screening after finding a low percent of healthcare workers had a positive TB test at baseline and follow up testing. The new recommendations still include baseline testing for preemployment. Also there should be ongoing evaluation if either the test is positive or if symptoms appear in a person without a history of TB or latent TB. Encourage persons with symptoms to be evaluated. However in the absence of exposure or documented transmission no further testing is required. The recommendations for two step testing have not changed. The two step process is designed to determine if infection is present in someone with waning immunity. It is recommended that HCP with untreated latent TB have a symptoms evaluation/screening every year. Treatment and follow would be determined by those results. Education on an annual basis should be provided. For updated information please see www.tbcontrollers.org

Source: Tuberculosis Screening, Testing, and Treatment of U.S. Health Care Personnel: Recommendations from the National Tuberculosis Controllers Association and CDC, 2019

Weekly / May 17, 2019 / 68(19);439–443

In general, persons not receiving treatment who have or are suspected of having pulmonary or laryngeal TB should be considered infectious if they are coughing, undergoing cough-inducing or aerosol-generating procedures, or have sputum smears positive for acid-fast bacilli. Persons with extrapulmonary TB are not considered infectious unless they have concomitant pulmonary disease, nonpulmonary disease located in the respiratory tract or oral cavity, or extrapulmonary disease that includes an open abscess or lesion. Co-infection with HIV does not appear to affect the infectiousness of TB patients.

Goal

The primary goal is to be able to identify and isolate a person with active or suspected TB. This measure will reduce the risk of transmission to staff or patients. You would not be expected to diagnose TB, but you should be trained to recognize the signs and symptoms of disease. Your written TB control plan should include policies, education, training, and standard operating procedures based upon

Risk classifications for health-care settings that serve communities with high incidence of tuberculosis (TB) and recommended frequency of screening for *Mycobacterium tuberculosis* infection among health-care workers (HCWs)*

| Setting | Risk classification[†] | | Potential ongoing transmission[§] |
	Low risk	Medium risk	
Inpatient <200 beds	<3 TB patients/year	≥3 TB patients/year	Evidence of ongoing *M. tuberculosis* transmission, regardless of setting
Inpatient ≥200 beds	<6 TB patients/year	≥6 TB patients/year	
Outpatient; and nontraditional facility-based	<3 TB patients/year	≥3 TB patients/year	
TB treatment facilities	Settings in which • persons who will be treated have been demonstrated to have latent TB infection (LTBI) and not TB disease • a system is in place to promptly detect and triage persons who have signs or symptoms of TB disease to a setting in which persons with TB disease are treated • no cough-inducing or aerosol-generating procedures are performed	Settings in which • persons with TB disease are encountered • criteria for low risk are not otherwise met	
Laboratories	Laboratories in which clinical specimens that might contain *M. tuberculosis* are not manipulated	Laboratories in which clinical specimens that might contain *M. tuberculosis* might be manipulated	

Recommendations for Screening Frequency

	Low risk	Medium risk	Potential ongoing transmission
Baseline two-step TST or one BAMT[¶]	Yes, for all HCWs upon hire	Yes, for all HCWs upon hire	Yes, for all HCWs upon hire
Serial TST or BAMT screening of HCWs	No**	At least every 12 months[††]	As needed in the investigation of potential ongoing transmission[§§]
TST or BAMT for HCWs upon unprotected exposure to *M. tuberculosis*	Perform a contact investigation (i.e., administer one TST or BAMT as soon as possible at the time of exposure, and, if the result is negative, give a second test [TST or BAMT, whichever was used for the first test] 8–10 weeks after the end of exposure to *M. tuberculosis*)[¶¶]		

* The term Health-care workers (HCWs) refers to all paid and unpaid persons working in health-care settings who have the potential for exposure to *M. tuberculosis* through air space shared with persons with TB disease.

† Settings that serve communities with a high incidence of TB disease or that treat populations at high risk (e.g., those with human immunodeficiency virus infection or other immunocompromising conditions) or that treat patients with drug-resistant TB disease might need to be classified as medium risk, even if they meet the low-risk criteria.

§ A classification of potential ongoing transmission should be applied to a specific group of HCWs or to a specific area of the health-care setting in which evidence of ongoing transmission is apparent, if such a group or area can be identified. Otherwise, a classification of potential ongoing transmission should be applied to the entire setting. This classification should be temporary and warrants immediate investigation and corrective steps after a determination has been made that ongoing transmission has ceased. The setting should be reclassified as medium risk, and the recommended timeframe for this medium risk classification is at least 1 year.

¶ All HCWs upon hire should have a documented baseline two-step tuberculin skin test (TST) or one blood assay for *M. tuberculosis* (BAMT) result at each new health-care setting, even if the setting is determined to be low risk. In certain settings, a choice might be made to not perform baseline TB screening or serial TB screening for HCWs who 1) will never be in contact with or have shared air space with patients who have TB disease (e.g., telephone operators who work in a separate building from patients) or 2) will never be in contact with clinical specimens that might contain *M. tuberculosis*. Establishment of a reliable baseline result can be beneficial if subsequent screening is needed after an unexpected exposure to *M. tuberculosis*.

** HCWs in settings classified as low risk do not need to be included in the serial TB screening program.

†† The frequency of screening for infection with *M. tuberculosis* will be determined by the risk assessment for the setting and determined by the Infection Control team.

§§ During an investigation of potential ongoing transmission of *M. tuberculosis*, testing for *M. tuberculosis* infection should be performed every 8–10 weeks until a determination has been made that ongoing transmission has ceased. Then the setting should be reclassified as medium risk for at least 1 year.

¶¶ Procedures for contact investigations should not be confused with two-step TSTs, which are used for baseline TST results for newly hired HCWs.

CDC. Guidelines for Preventing the Transmission of *Mycobacterium tuberculosis* in Health-Care Settings, 2005 www.cdc.gov/tb/publications/guidelines/list_date.htm

the results of the risk assessment. Office policies should include how to identify persons with active TB, where to refer them to medical care, where to refer them for urgent dental care, education, counseling and training of staff, and periodic tuberculin skin testing according to current CDC recommendations.

Considerations for Dental Treatment

Patient medical history forms and patient health history interviews should include questions regarding history of TB and signs and symptoms of possible infection. If a patient is suspected of having active TB, isolate the patient from other patients and ask them to wear a surgical mask or otherwise cover their mouth and nose while in your office. Patients should not remain in the office any longer than is necessary to evaluate their dental condition and be appropriately referred. Routine dental care should be deferred until a patient is no longer infectious as determined by their primary care provider and communicated to your office. If urgent dental care is needed, patients should be referred to an appropriate dental facility that has airborne infection control measures in place such as environmental controls and personal respiratory protection. TB infection control measures may include an isolation room, areas of negative pressure, or HEPA filtration for circulating air. Standard surgical masks do not protect against TB transmission. Respiratory protection such as a properly fitted, FDA-cleared N-95 personal respirator should be used if performing dental treatment.

Dental procedures are capable of stimulating coughing and the spread of infectious particles. The generation of droplet nuclei containing TB has not been demonstrated as a result of dental treatment, but the possibility may exist. Patients and DHCP share the same air space over time and this could contribute to TB transmission.

If you or another staff member is suspected of having active TB then a prompt medical evaluation is necessary. You should not return to work until a diagnosis of TB has been ruled out by a healthcare professional. If active TB is diagnosed, then a return to work would be indicated only after successful therapy and with approval from the HCP.

Other Airborne Considerations

Organisms transmitted through the air may lead to upper respiratory infections such as the common cold, flu/influenza and pneumonia.

Airborne considerations for dentistry are not limited to infectious diseases. Indoor air quality and its association with upper respiratory diseases is being studied by a variety of scientists. These diseases under investigation include not only infections diseases but also noninfectious diseases such as occupationally acquired asthma.

Dental Unit Waterlines (DUWL) delivers water for cooling and irrigation to the dental handpieces, sonic and ultrasonic scalers, air/water syringes and other devices used in patient care. Biofilms form on the inner walls of the small-bore plastic tubing in dental unit water lines (DUWL). The microorganisms isolated from the DUWL are primarily of naturally occurring, slime-producing bacteria and fungi. If the biofilm growth in the DUWL is not controlled, microbial contamination in effluent water may exceed 1,000,000 colony forming units per milliliter (CFU/mL) of water. (See Course 4 pages 9-11 for Dental Unit Waterline Treatment information)

Most microorganisms recovered from dental unit waterlines (DUWLs) occur naturally in aquatic environments. Dental unit waterlines colonized with gram negative heterotrophic biofilms can have high levels of lipopolysaccharide (LPS also known as endotoxin) that can trigger and/or exacerbate asthma in dental patients and dental healthcare personnel (DHCP). LPS can also cause skin rashes, gastrointestinal reactions and may result in delayed wound healing.

Opportunistic human pathogens in DUWLs, such as *Pseudomonas aeruginosa,* nontuberculous mycobacteria (NTM) and *Legionella* species have also been found. Exposure to contaminated procedural water most likely led to two cases of postoperative *Pseudomonas* infections in immunocompromised patients.

Two outbreaks of pediatric postoperative infections in Georgia and California were the result of *Mycobacterium abscessus* exposure isolated from DUWLs.

In 2014, a fatal case of *Legionella* pneumonia in an elderly woman in Italy was traced to the identical *Legionella* species found in the DUWLs of the dental practice where the patient had received recent treatment. A 2017 a Swedish case report described another fatal case of Legionellosis in an elderly immunocompromised man who received dental treatment in a hospital dental clinic.

Serological evidence of exposure to *Legionella* bacteria have been reported in dental health-care personnel. A post-hoc review of screening for serologic markers of *Legionella* exposure in dentists conducted as part of the American Dental Association (ADA) dentist health screening program however, found that dentists appeared to be no more likely to exhibit evidence of exposure than the general population.

Source: Dental Unit Water Quality: Organization for Safety, Asepsis and Prevention White Paper and Recommendations – 2018 published in the *Journal of Dental Infection Control and Safety* Volume 1/Issue 1, provides more detail on the background of dental unit water quality as well as recommendations. To read the full article, visit: osapjdics.scholasticahq.com

One of the best ways to reduce the risk of occupational exposures is to determine where, how, and which employees are at risk. The Infection Control Coordinator or Safety Officer should identify job procedures and tasks that pose a risk for occupational exposure incidents. The Coordinator should also identify which employees perform these procedures in order to assure that they are:

1. **Trained specifically to carry out those procedures, including Standard Precautions and Work Practice Controls.**
2. **Provided with the appropriate Personal Protective Equipment and Engineering Controls.**
3. **Offered the HBV immunization series.**
4. **Offered any other appropriate protection, training, etc.**

Example:

If you operate a sterilizer, you must know the associated procedures of the sterilizer and the proper handling of the instruments. If you work only in an operatory and are never involved in cleanup, you may not need to be trained specifically in the operation of a sterilizer. However, in either case you would need to be given instruction about bloodborne pathogens and be aware of the recommendation to receive the hepatitis B immunization.

Exposure Risk Determination

OSHA requires that each employee's potential for occupational exposure be documented in the office's Infection Control/Exposure Control Plan. For example, according to the Bloodborne Pathogens Standard, you either have the potential for exposure to bloodborne pathogens, or you do not have potential exposure. All personnel involved in clinical care or in the handling or management of the dental operatory, instruments, dental laboratory materials, dental waste, etc. are considered to have potential exposure to bloodborne pathogens.

Determine Exposure Risk Without PPE

When an exposure risk determination is made, it is *without* consideration to any PPE the employee may use. Although PPE items are excellent barriers to infection, they can have limitations due to improper use, fit, failure, or possible flaws. Learning to use the proper procedures, *together* with PPE, is your best protection against exposure incidents.

Please find the written Infection Control/Exposure Control Plan for your practice before proceeding with this section.

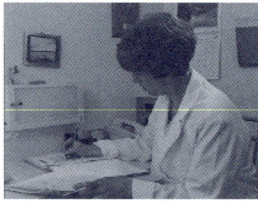

FAMILIARIZE YOURSELF WITH ITS CONTENTS

Your potential for exposure must be documented in the Infection Control/Exposure Control Plan. It is the responsibility of your employer to assess your occupational risk. This assessment determines your need for training, indications for immunizations and health assessments, selection of PPE, standard operating procedures (SOPs) to be followed, and types of records required.

Note:

Temporary Workers and Independent Contractors: These individuals must comply with OSHA regulations when they work in your office, just like all employees. The supplying employer and the using employer have a shared responsibility to ensure that workers are protected from workplace hazards. Their training, HBV immunizations and Postexposure Management are the responsibility of the supplying employer (themselves, if an independent contractor). Contracts that address these issues are recommended so that all parties fully understand where their responsibilities lie.

Depending on the type of work, all employees may need some level of training. In a dental office, employers may recognize the need to treat all employees as if there is a potential for exposure. Likewise, students in an educational program should also receive appropriate training for both their on and off-site clinical settings.

Example:

Betty, the office manager, works only at the front desk managing the waiting room, answering the telephone, making appointments, and performing other clerical tasks. She is in her late 50s, is in excellent health, enjoys what she does, and is never involved in clinical tasks. She has not been trained in dental infection control and safety and has never been immunized against HBV.

One day, the dental assistant and dental hygienist were away from the office when there was a full patient schedule. For the first and only time, Betty was asked to assist the dentist and did so without wearing the appropriate PPE.

A month later she developed infectious mononucleosis, even though she did not have any of the normal risk factors. A teenage patient, who was treated the same day that Betty was required to assist the dentist, was later diagnosed with infectious mononucleosis.

In this circumstance, common sense would dictate that this employee should never have been asked to assist in the first place. Betty had neither the training, nor the necessary experience. However, if this situation could have been anticipated, she could have received all the appropriate training, HBV immunizations and PPE.

List four tasks that you perform and indicate whether or not each has a risk of an exposure incident:

Task	Risk?
_____	yes no
_____	yes no
_____	yes no
_____	yes no

Primary: Preventing an Exposure Incident

The primary emphasis is to prevent an exposure incident from ever occurring. This can be accomplished by using appropriate techniques, and safe dental devices. However, in spite of your best efforts, injuries may still occur. Treating and containing an injury as soon as possible (ASAP) is critical and therefore, each employer must have a postexposure plan with specific procedures in place, called the Postexposure Management Plan. This plan should contain detailed, step-by-step instructions, mandated by OSHA and recommended by the USPHS, for managing exposure incidents. A discussion with a Worker's Compensation carrier should include procedures to be followed and forms to be filed.

As part of the Postexposure Management Plan, each employer should select and identify a designated healthcare provider experienced with occupational exposures and current USPHS recommendations for postexposure management who will provide medical follow-up with a given copy of the Bloodborne Pathogens Standard, a description of employees' job duties, the assurance that in the case of an incident, the employer will provide documentation on the incident and written informed consent as necessary. The informed consent form should contain at least the following:
1 · The nature of the test to be performed
2 · The benefits and risks of testing
3 · Alternatives and their benefits and risks
4 · The exact limits of confidentiality

Prior to an incident, employers should consider when an exposure incident may be covered by Workers' Compensation. A discussion with a Workers' Compensation carrier should include procedures to be followed and forms to be filed.

Secondary: Managing an Exposure Incident

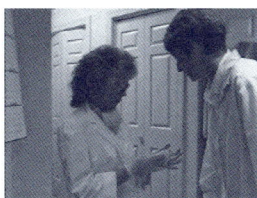

An occupational exposure is considered an urgent medical concern that demands immediate action. After an exposure, there are several steps that *must be taken immediately* to minimize the extent of an injury or risk of disease transmission. This is basic first aid. While detailed procedures are outlined in your Postexposure Management Plan, the single most important element to effectively handle an exposure incident is to take immediate action. Do not under any circumstance hesitate or ignore the incident.

Basic First Aid: Postexposure Incident Containment Steps
1 · **Treat and contain the injury**
   a) **Infectious** - Cleanse the exposed area as indicated (see note on the next page)
   b) **Chemical** - Wash or flush affected areas if indicated on the Safety Data Sheet
   c) **Physical** - Use approved first aid procedures

2 · **Immediately notify the Infection Control Coordinator or Safety Officer or senior employee**

3 · **Get the Infection Control/Exposure Control Plan and follow the appropriate plan**
   Tab A: Infection Postexposure Management Plan
   Tab B: Chemical Postexposure Management Plan
   Tab C: Physical Postexposure Management Plan
Note on Infectious Exposure Incident: Includes any eye, mouth, mucus membrane, nonintact skin, or other parenteral contact with blood or other potentially infectious material.
Percutaneous (puncture wounds): wash with soap and water and control bleeding
Mucous membrane (splashes to the nose or mouth): Flush with water
Splashes to eyes: irrigate with clean water, saline, or sterile solution
Splashes to nonintact skin: wash with soap and water

Use of antiseptics for wound care or squeezing the wound will not reduce the risk of HIV transmission. The use of bleach or disinfectants is not recommended.

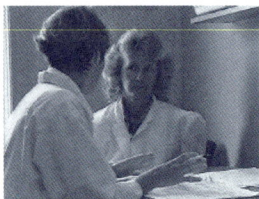

After containing the injury and applying initial first aid, your Infection Control Coordinator or Safety Officer or employer will begin the process of postexposure management and follow-up as indicated in the Infection Control/Exposure Control Plan. Although all three Postexposure Management Plans (Tabs A, B, and C) contain similar steps, each has specific medical follow-up procedures related to the source of the exposure: blood or other body fluid, chemical or physical. Unlike chemical or physical incidents where medical follow-up is determined by the agent or injury, medical follow-up for infectious exposure is in accordance with USPHS recommendations and as required by OSHA. The following describes the medical management of blood exposures.

Medical Evaluation and Intervention

When an exposure occurs, the exposed DHCP should be put in immediate contact with the designated healthcare provider (HCP). It is important to do this quickly because the HCP may recommend a post-exposure treatment that should start as soon as possible. For example, treatment with antiretroviral drugs after exposure to HIV-infected blood, known as post-exposure prophylaxis (PEP), should start as soon as possible within 72 hours of the exposure.

The HCP will assess the nature of the injury and determine which baseline tests are indicated. In addition, a review of employee and source patient information (if known) will determine the course of medical treatment. If the dental patient (also called the source, source patient or source person) is available and agrees to do so, he or she should be tested by the HCP for bloodborne diseases. Certain circumstances may require the immediate (ideally within 2 hours) use of postexposure prophylaxis with antiretroviral agents in accordance with the most current USPHS guidelines. Employees should also be instructed to report any illness to the HCP for possible association with HIV, HBV and/or HCV infection.

Counseling is a necessary component of Postexposure Management and is especially required when baseline testing is indicated. Counseling should include a discussion on the nature of testing, results, and about the protection of personal contacts from the transmission of disease. Blood may be collected and tested for HIV, HBV, and/or HCV for the employee and source patient with consent. In the case of HIV, the blood may be drawn and stored for 90 days before testing, giving a reluctant employee or source patient time to make an informed decision.

Note: All postexposure evaluations and HBV vaccination requirements must be made available to the employee at a reasonable time and place, and at no cost to the employee. Evaluations must be performed by a licensed physician or other appropriately licensed healthcare professional.

Evaluation of occupational exposure sources:
  Known sources
  · Test known sources for HBsAg, anti-ACV, and HIV antibody
    - Direct virus assays for routine screening of source patients are **not** recommended
    - Consider using a rapid HIV-antibody test
    - If the source person is **not** infected with a bloodborne pathogen, baseline testing or further follow-up of the exposed person is **not** necessary
  · For sources whose infection status remains unknown (e.g., the source person refuses testing), consider medical diagnoses, clinical symptoms or if the patient has reported risk factors to you, and history of risk behaviors.
  · Do not test discarded needles for bloodborne pathogens
  Unknown sources
  · For unknown sources, evaluate the likelihood of exposure to a source at high risk for infection
    - Consider likelihood of bloodborne pathogen infection among patients in the exposure setting

Hepatitis B Virus Postexposure Management

Vaccination and anti-body response status of exposed workers*	Treatment		
	Source HBsAg[1] Positive	Source HBsAg[1] Negative	Source unknown or not available for testing
Unvaccinated	HBIG[2] x 1 and initiate HB vaccine series[3]	Initiate HB vaccine series	Initiate HB vaccine series
Previously vaccinated			
Known responder[4]	No treatment	No treatment	No treatment
Known nonresponder[5]	HBIG x 1 and initiate revaccination or HBIG x 2 [6]	No treatment	If known high risk source, treat as if source were HBsAg-Positive Test exposed person for anti-HBs
Antibody response unknown	Test exposed person for anti-HBs[3] 1) If adequate,[4] no treatment is necessary 2) If inadequate,[5] administer HBIG x 1 and vaccine booster dose	No treatment	1) If adequate,[3] no treatment is necessary 2) If inadequate,[3] administer vaccine booster and recheck titer in 1-2 months

Reference: Updated U.S. Public Health Service Guidelines for the Management of Occupational Exposures to HBV, HCV, and HIV and Recommendations for Postexposure Prophylaxis, MMWR, 2001, Vol 50, No RR11;1-42

1 Hepatitis B surface antigen
2 Hepatitis B immune globulin; dose is 0.06 mL/kg intramuscularly
3 Hepatitis B vaccine
4 A responder is a person with adequate levels of serum antibody to HBsAg (i.e., anti-HBs >=10mIU/mL)
5 A nonresponder is a person with inadequate response to vaccination (i.e., serum anti-HBs < 10 mIU/mL)
6 The option of giving one dose of HBIG and reinitiating the vaccine series is preferred for nonresponders who have not completed a second 3-dose vaccine series. For persons who previously completed a second vaccine series but failed to respond, two doses of HBIG are preferred
7 Antibody to HBsAg
* Persons who have previously been infected with HBV are immune to reinfection and do not require postexposure prophylaxis.

Hepatitis C Virus Postexposure Management

There is no pre or post-exposure prophylaxis for HCV. A baseline test (anti-HCV) is recommended if there is concern that the patient may have hepatitis C. Medical follow-up consists of counseling, anti-HCV testing, liver function testing, and education on risk and prevention of secondary transmission. If HCV infection occurs in the exposed employee, there are now a variety of treatment options for early HCV infection.

HIV Postexposure Management

Occupational transmission of HIV to healthcare workers is extremely rare. However, for workers who are exposed, CDC has recommendations to minimize the risk of developing HIV. These recommendations also provide help in determining whether an exposed DHCP should receive PEP (antiretroviral medication taken after possible exposure to reduce the chance of infection with HIV) and in choosing the type of PEP regimen.

There are three important facts to consider in making a decision to take an anti-HIV drug after an exposure incident:

1) The average risk of HIV infection after all types of needlestick exposures to HIV-infected blood is 0.3%. However, the risk may be higher if the exposure involves a higher volume of blood, or if the patient is in the late stages of AIDS.

2) The risk of HIV infection after an occupational exposure may be reduced by postexposure prophylaxis with antiviral drugs.

3) Postexposure prophylaxis (PEP: the use of anti-HIV drugs) will not prevent all occupational infections nor will all exposures lead to infection.

HIV Postexposure Management (cont.)

Treatment of Exposed Worker When Source:		
Individual is positive for HIV infection, OR, Individual refused to be tested	Individual is tested and found seronegative and has no clinical manifestations of HIV infection	Individual cannot be identified
1) The exposed worker should be counseled about the risk of infection. 2) The exposed worker should be evaluated clinically and serologically for evidence of HIV infection as soon as possible after the exposure. 3) The exposed worker should be advised to seek and report medical evaluation for any febrile illness that occurs within 12 weeks after the exposure. 4) The exposed worker should be advised to refrain from blood donation and to use appropriate protection during sexual intercourse during the follow-up period, especially the first 6-12 weeks after exposure. An exposed worker who tests negative initially should be retested 6 weeks, 12 weeks, and a minimum of 6 months after exposure to determine whether transmission has occurred.	No further follow-up unless: 1) Evidence suggests that source may have been recently exposed. 2) Desire by worker or recommended by healthcare provider. If testing is done, the guidelines in the first column may be followed.	Decisions regarding appropriate follow-up should be individualized. Serologic testing should be done if the worker is concerned that HIV transmission may have occurred.

Reference: The information given in this table is based on recommendations from: Updated U.S. Public Health Service Guidelines for the Management of Occupational Exposures to HBV, HCV, and HIV and Recommendations for Postexposure Prophylaxis, MMWR, 2001, Vol 50, No RR11;1-42

See Updated U.S. Public Health Service Guidelines for the Management of Occupational Exposures to HIV and Recommendations for Postexposure Prophylaxis. Infect Control Hosp Epidemiol. 2013 Sep;34(9):875-92. stacks.cdc.gov/view/cdc/20711
Additional Resource: www.cdc.gov/hiv/basics/pep.html

For additional assistance, you can contact the PEPline at the University of California, San Francisco. PEPline offers online information or phone consultation for urgent exposure management.

Online:

nccc.ucsf.edu/clinician-consultation/pep-post-exposure-prophylaxis/

Phone Consultation: (888) 448-4911

Ongoing Medical Follow-Up

Ongoing medical follow-up of an exposed employee includes counseling, evaluation of reported illnesses, monitoring of treatment and, possibly, additional testing. All must be accomplished in a confidential manner. This does not give the employer authority to be informed of the results of the source patient or the exposed employee's test results.

Information available to the employer only relates to whether or not a HBV immunization was indicated and given – all other information is between the HCP and the employee. Since state laws are not consistent, you may wish to contact your state's Attorney General's office, Board of Registration in Dentistry, your local association, or malpractice carrier. However, the employer must inform the exposed employee of all the applicable laws or regulations that protect the source patient's confidentiality.

The confidentiality of patient information has always been a cornerstone of the medical and dental professions and should be respected.

Tertiary: Lessons to be Learned

Once the exposure incident has been managed, the last step is to review the entire situation. All steps should be taken to determine how the incident occurred in order to reduce future risks. The goal is to keep that type of exposure and anything similar from occurring again.

Recommended steps for tertiary prevention include:
- **Evaluate the circumstances of incident, including devices or equipment used**
- **Review policies, procedures, products, and practices**
- **Review manufacturers' directions for all products and devices**
- **Review and update written plans as indicated**
- **Review incident reports:**
  - Evaluate the circumstances
  - Identify ways to prevent a similar situation
- **Discuss appropriate modifications with staff including specific training and consideration of alternative devices.**

Employee Records

All employee medical records must be kept confidential for the duration of employment and for 30 years thereafter. These records may be kept by the employer or may be kept by the designated HCP. If a practice is sold, either the original employer or the new employer is required to maintain the records. If a practice is to be terminated, the employer must either maintain the records or notify OSHA. OSHA may require that the records be turned over to them. These records are covered in Course #7.

Exposure Control Plan

When required, a written plan, specific to your office, should be created outlining step-by-step procedures to be followed in the event of an exposure incident or emergency. It should be available in a central location for quick reference and should start with management of the injury, and list the local phone numbers of physicians, hospitals and ambulance services. This plan should be placed in your Infection Control/Exposure Control Plan or binder. All employees must be trained to this plan.

Where is your Postexposure Plan located?

_____

What is the name of your practice's designated healthcare provider or facility?

_____

In the event of an incident, who would you inform?

_____

Who is your Infection Control Coordinator or Safety Officer?

_____

Now that you have learned the basics of Postexposure Management, please find your office's Infection Control/Exposure Control Plan and turn to the section where the Postexposure Management Plans are located and review the plans.

Sharps Safety and the Needlestick Prevention Act

Mandated by the Needlestick Safety and Prevention Act, changes to the Occupational Safety & Health Administration's (OSHA) Bloodborne Pathogens Standard were published January 18, 2001, and were effective April 18, 2001. The revisions clarify the need for employers, including dental employers, to select safer sharps* devices as they become available and to involve non-managerial employees involved in direct patient care in identifying and choosing the devices. To demonstrate compliance, employers must document solicitation of input from employees in the written Exposure Control Plan.

For dental applications, such devices would include safety needles, and/or safety syringes, safety scalpels and sutures, and needleless IV catheters, ports, and injection systems.

Dental practices should consider assessing sharps safety devices a two-step process:
1. Screening devices
2. Evaluating devices

Screening

Screening helps staff make decisions about clinical and safety considerations before bringing a safety device into the patient-care setting. It consists of reviewing product literature and information to identify new and possibly safer devices that are available, physically examining the safety device, comparing it to the device currently used in your practice, and measuring it against the criteria that has been established as important.

A representative dentist, hygienist or assistant who will be handling the device should participate in the screening phase. It is important that each person involved in the screening process has a sample of the device as well as the device currently in use in your office.

A form can be used to collect the opinions and observations of staff about a new safety device. Once all personnel involved in the screening phase have completed the screening form, they should discuss the results among themselves and with the Infection Control Coordinator or Safety Officer or their employer to determine whether to proceed to the next phase – evaluating the device in your clinic setting.

After a device passes the screening phase it should be scheduled for evaluation in your clinic setting. The evaluation phase always includes a pilot test in an actual clinic setting. New safety devices that have not been screened to make sure that they meet clinical, staff- and patient-safety should not be used on a patient.

A representative dentist, hygienist or assistant who will be using or handling the device should be included in the pilot test portion of the evaluation phase. A form can be used to collect the opinions, observations and reactions of staff who are pilot testing the new safety dental device.

Steps for Conducting a Pilot Test in the Evaluation Phase

1. Staff receive training on correct use of the device.
2. Staff use the safety device and document their experience through informal feedback and by completing an evaluation form.
3. The employer or the Infection Control Coordinator or Safety Officer monitors whether the device is being used properly, and stops the pilot test if the device is found to be unsafe.
4. At the end of the pilot test discussions should be held with staff members who were involved in the test and completed the evaluation forms to determine the criteria that should receive the most consideration.
5. Findings are reviewed by the employer and Infection Control Coordinator or Safety Officer and a decision is made about continuing to use the new device in the practice.

Forms used for screening and evaluating safer sharps should be kept in the written Exposure Control Plan as documentation of the OSHA mandate that requires employers to select safer sharps devices as they become available and to involve employees in identifying and choosing the devices.

Sample Forms

Sample sharps screening and evaluation forms are available from the CDC and can downloaded at the following link:
www.cdc.gov/oralhealth/infectioncontrol/forms.html

An additional resource from CDC is the *Workbook for Designing, Implementing, and Evaluating a Sharps Injury Prevention Program*
www.cdc.gov/sharpssafety/pdf/sharpsworkbook_2008.pdf

OSHA Regulations

www.cdc.gov/oralhealth/infectioncontrol/forms.htm
www.osha.gov/SLTC/bloodbornepathogens/index.html

In addition to the training requirements of OSHA's Bloodborne Pathogens Standard, a copy of the standard is required to be made available to all DCHP. This OSHA document, 29 CFR Part 1910.1030, Bloodborne Pathogens, may be located in your Infection Control/Exposure Control Plan or at another location in the office. We recommend that you ask your Infection Control Coordinator or Safety Officer where the Bloodborne Pathogens Standard is located and, within the next few weeks, look over this standard. As a DCHP, you are required to be familiar with those parts of the standard that apply to your job and procedures at your place of employment.

For more detailed information, an excellent resource is at the OSHA website at www.osha.gov.

Where is your practice's copy of OSHA's Bloodborne Pathogens Standard located?

Discussion

Below are some questions that will assist you in a discussion with your Infection Control Coordinator or Safety Officer.

The post-test for course #2 is in the back of this book. Take the test and use it to discuss what you've learned with your Infection control coordinator or safety officer.

You have now completed the workbook segment for Course #2. Below are some sample questions that will also assist you in your discussion with your Infection Control Coordinator or Safety Officer, employer, or dentist, and other staff members.

Question: *What is the risk to office staff of being exposed to HIV when handling patient records?*

Answer: There is a risk of contamination from spatter, aerosolization of blood and body fluids, or contact with treatment gloves and equipment in the dental operatory. For that reason, patient records should *never* be in close proximity to clinical activities. If this work practice control is observed, the chances of transmitting HIV through patient records is virtually zero. It should be noted that blood containing HIV only survives outside the body while wet, and for a period of a half hour or less at room temperature. In addition, in this situation the virus can only be transmitted through an open wound or sore in the staff worker. It is unlikely for all these conditions to exist at once.

Question: *Can I see my own doctor if I have an exposure incident?*

Answer: Yes, but you and your employer should discusses specific issues, regulations and guidelines for postexposure management with your doctor and ensure that he/she understands the Bloodborne Pathogens Standard *prior to an incident occurring.* Your own doctor may not be familiar with Bloodborne Pathogens transmissions or the most current USPHS/CDC recommendations for exposure management.

It may be more efficient and convenient for your employer to contract with a single healthcare provider who will be responsible for postexposure management and incident follow-up. Any such arrangements should be discussed with all employees. The HCP must be provided or be familiar with the guidelines for exposure incident management and medical follow-up.

Notes

Objectives

Upon completion of this course on personal protection, you will be able to:

1. Explain the type of protection provided by each of the following:
   - Protective eyewear
   - Facemasks
   - Gloves
   - Barrier attire
   - Face shields
2. Compare and contrast the benefits and limitations of five personal protective barriers (5 types of PPE).
3. Explain the concept of procedure specific PPE.
4. Identify three antiseptic agents used in your or a dental office.
5. Differentiate handwashing and surgical hand antisepsis.
6. Demonstrate an effective handwashing technique.
7. Demonstrate a surgical hand antisepsis.

Focus

The last time you had a cold or flu, did you know how you got it? Between the time you were infected and then felt ill, do you know how many people *you* exposed?

Infections

We are in constant contact with pathogens, organisms that are capable of causing disease. Since they are everywhere, contact with them is unavoidable:
- **Someone sneezes in line at the grocery store**
- **You are in an elevator and someone coughs**
- **You kiss your child good night**

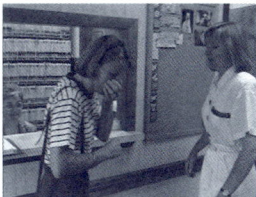

Any of these everyday scenarios, and others like them, can result in the transmission of disease, and we accept the presence of common non-life-threatening diseases as a fact of daily life. We understand that their transmission primarily occurs by the mouth and the nose, and we rarely take any precautions against them. The hands are the most common mechanism of transporting contamination.

More serious pathogens exist, however, that are transmitted through unprotected contact with blood and other serum body fluids. Examples are HBV, HCV, and HIV, which are diseases that can cause serious illness and death. (see Course #2)

Other Hazards

The use of barriers is not just for protection from infectious agents. Your office uses a wide array of chemicals for patient treatment, X-rays, lab work, cleaning, disinfection and sterilization, which become additional hazards in the workplace. Toxic and other irritating chemicals can be found in the form of solutions, vapors or as residue. Some are easily identifiable, while other chemicals may be invisible or odorless and can present a danger, even if properly used. Adequate protection is necessary to prevent injury related to contact with chemicals.

You have an obligation and a responsibility to prevent the transfer of infectious agents or microorganisms to patients, and to protect them from chemical and physical hazards. You also have an obligation to protect yourself. Consequently, you must create an environment that places barriers between you, the environment, and others. *These barriers, along with other exposure control precautions, must be used for all patients during all clinical procedures,* or *"everything for everyone."*

Standard Precautions

This concept is called *Standard Precautions* and is the first tier of precautions to prevent the transmission of infections. Standard Precautions integrate and expand the elements of universal precautions (consider all blood and body fluids as infectious) into a standard of care designed to protect the dental team and patients from pathogens that can be spread by blood or any other body fluid, nonintact skin and mucous membranes.

Transmission-Based Precautions

Transmission-based precautions are a second tier of precautions that are added to standard precautions when disease transmission cannot be completely interrupted by standard precautions alone. These infection prevention and control precautions are for the care of patients who are infected or colonized with highly contagious pathogens spread through airborne, droplet, or contact routes. Transmission-based precautions consist of standard precautions, plus precautions specific to how the specific pathogen is transmitted. Outbreaks of emerging and re-emerging disease occur, some requiring transmission-based precautions. In the case of an outbreak it is important to have correct and credible information to determine action. CDC is an appropriate resource for this information. More information and a detailed list of transmission based precautions can be accessed on the CDC website at:

www.cdc.gov/hicpac/pdf/isolation/Isolation2007.pdf
www.cdc.gov/hicpac/2007IP/2007ip_appendA.html
Executive Summary:
   www.cdc.gov/hicpac/2007IP/2007ip_ExecSummary.html

Examples include:

- ## Contact Precautions
  - Methicillin-resistant *Staphylococcus aureus* (MRSA).
    MRSA is a type of bacteria that is referred to as a multi-drug resistant organism (MDRO). MDROs are bacteria and other microorganisms that are resistant to one or more kind of antimicrobial drug. Sometimes these are called "superbugs" because they are very difficult to kill. In healthcare settings, MRSA most often is spread indirectly from patient to patient through contact from contaminated hands of healthcare workers. Hand hygiene is very important to limit spread of infection between patients. Learn more about MRSA skin infections at: Methicillin-resistant *Staphylococcus aureus* (MRSA) Resource: Klevens, et al: "jada.ada.org/article/S0002-8177(14)65410-6/abstract" Learn more about MRSA skin infections at: www.cdc.gov/mrsa/mrsa_initiative/skin_infection/mrsa_faqs.html

- **Droplet Precautions**
  - o Chickenpox/Varicella Zoster
    Chickenpox, caused by the varicella-zoster virus, is a disease that causes blisters, often with severe itching. Chickenpox is very contagious and spreads easily through coughing and sneezing, but can also spread by touching or breathing in the virus from the blisters. CDC provides detailed information about chickenpox at: www.cdc.gov/chickenpox/about/index.html

  - o Flu/Influenza
    CDC provides detailed information about the current flu season and recommended seasonal flu vaccine. CDC also provides information about different kinds of flu, such as avian influenza, swine flu, and pandemic influenza. Visit the CDC flu website at: www.cdc.gov/flu/

- **Airborne Precautions**
  - o Tuberculosis (TB)
    TB is caused by a bacterium known as *Mycobacterium tuberculosis*. TB spreads from one person to another through the air when an infected person with TB of the lungs or throat coughs, sneezes, talks, sings. This sends TB bacteria into the air where they can be breathed in by others nearby and cause infection. Detailed information about TB can be found at the CDC website: www.cdc.gov/tb/default.htm

    Additional Resources:
    Cleveland JL, Robison VA, Panlilio AL. Tuberculosis Epidemiology, Diagnosis and Infection Control Recommendations for Dental Settings. An Update on the Centers for Disease Control and Prevention Guidelines. jada.ada.org/article/S0002-8177(14)64527-X/abstract

    Merte JL et al. An epidemiologic investigation of occupational transmission of *Mycobacterium tuberculosis* infection to dental health care personnel. jada.ada.org/article/S0002-8177(14)60040-4/pdf

Personal Protection Consists of Barriers and Other Exposure Control Precautions

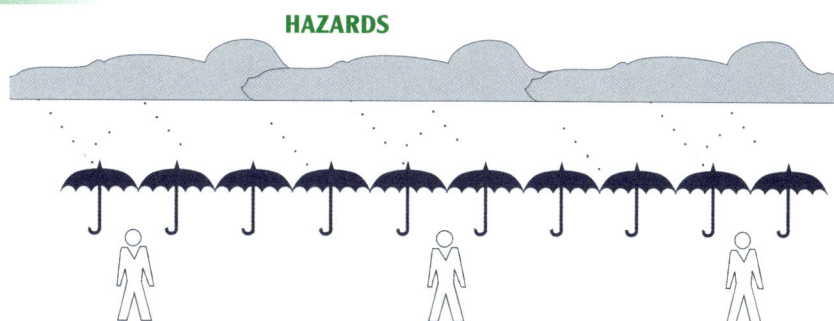

HAZARDS

The rationale for barriers against infectious agents is straightforward. Many people who carry infectious disease show no symptoms, are unaware that they are infected, and have no idea that their blood, saliva, or respiratory secretions may be capable of transmitting infectious diseases. Therefore, it must be assumed that *all* patients, *all* providers, and *all* body fluids are potential transmitters of infectious agents, and are potential sources for contamination (passing of infectious agents from one person to another). Consequently, you will encounter the following situations:

1 · **Patients who are unaware that they are infected and that their blood and/or saliva is capable of transmitting infectious agents**

2 · **Patients who do not wish to reveal a known infectious disease**

3 · **Patients who, based on provided information or physical assessment, are assumed to be healthy**

Even if you know the patient well, you can not assume that he or she is presently free of infectious disease or will remain so upon subsequent visits. You also cannot rely on information from a medical history questionaire to determine if a patient is infectious, as medical histories are limited to the information a patient knows or is willing to share.

Respiratory Hygiene/Cough Etiquette

When patients are sick, or are accompanied by persons who are sick, they can spread infection to others in the waiting area, restrooms, front desk or other parts of your dental facility. Respiratory Hygiene/Cough Etiquette, an important part of standard precautions, applies to any patient or staff member who shows signs of respiratory illness such as a cough, congestion or runny nose. Your dental practice should have a system in place to detect and manage potentially infectious persons soon after they arrive at your facility. Your infection control program should include a plan to:

- Teach staff:
  - the importance of preventing the spread of respiratory germs.
  - to identify people who have signs and symptoms of a respiratory infection, beginning at entry to your facility and during the entire visit.
  - the importance of ways to prevent the spread of respiratory germs from patients with signs and symptoms of a respiratory infection.
- Post signs with instructions to:
  - cover mouth/nose when coughing or sneezing.
  - use and properly discard tissues.
  - clean hands after coming in contact with respiratory secretions.
- Provide:
  - tissues and no-touch trash bins.
  - resources for hand hygiene in or near waiting areas.
  - or offer masks to people with a runny nose, cough or other signs of respiratory illness when they enter your facility.

You may or may not know the infectious status of yourself, a patient, or the materials you are handling, or the exact nature or toxicity of a chemical. Therefore, it is necessary to use Standard Precautions and possibly additional precautions to protect yourself. While all risks cannot be eliminated, your goal is to *reduce* these risks as much as possible.

What is your definition of Standard Precautions?

_____

_____

_____

_____

Personal Protection

There are two methods to prevent you from becoming infected with a disease. The first is your body's protection which combats disease *after* exposure and includes your natural immune system, reinforced by immunization. The second method is the use of *physical barrier protection*, which prevents the transmission of, or exposure to, infectious agents, through the use of your Personal Protective Equipment (PPE).

Hepatitis B and Other Immunizations

Immunization is the most effective tool against certain diseases, including: influenza, mumps, rubeola, rubella, tetanus, and hepatitis B. The CDC recommends that healthcare workers review and update their childhood vaccination series on a regular basis. It is important to follow CDC's most current recommendations for adult immunizations. The CDC and OSAP websites carry the most up-to-date information (cdc.gov or osap.org).

Do You Know Your Immunization Status for the Following Diseases? (Circle Answers)

You may want to follow-up with your physician if you are unsure of your status. It would also be advisable to note the last date of immunization.

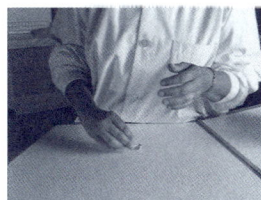

Hepatitis B	YES	NO	**Rubella (German Measles)**	YES	NO
Hepatitis A	YES	NO	**Rubeola (Measles)**	YES	NO
Mumps	YES	NO	**Tetanus**	YES	NO
Polio	YES	NO	**Influenza (yearly)**	YES	NO
Pneumonia	YES	NO	**Varicella (Chicken Pox, Shingles)**	YES	NO

If you are working with patients who are immigrants from areas with endemic (native) diseases, or you are treating patients from known high risk groups, you may be at increased risk. In these and similar situations you should evaluate the risk and receive immunizations in addition to the required HBV vaccination (see previous table). For example, if a dental practice is in a community that had a recent outbreak of measles, all employees may be advised to determine their level of protection and, if necessary, update their measles immunizations. Dental facilities should have a written policy within their Infection Control/Exposure Control Plan, including the protocol to for treating all patients, even those who have not been vaccinated for vaccine preventable diseases such as Measles.

Personal Protective Equipment

Immunizations are not available against all diseases. A second line of defense is to create *physical* barriers between yourself and disease-producing organisms or hazardous substances. These barriers are called Personal Protective Equipment (PPE) and in the dental setting include gloves, masks or face shields, eyewear, and protective clothing (gowns, laboratory coats, uniforms, etc.).

Note

It is wise to offer patients some form of protective eyewear, either their own glasses or sunglasses, or a pair of inexpensive, reusable eyewear supplied by your office and washed between patients (see Course #5).

Procedure-Specific PPE

In general, your everyday PPE is well defined; however, there are times that the selection of additional PPE must be made based on the exposure or potential for exposure for each procedure – not on the patient's possible infectious state. So, *PPE is standard for the procedure regardless of the patient* – "Everything for everyone for all procedures." For example, when ultrasonic scaling is performed, there is increased aerosolization, so a face shield might be worn over the mask and a disposable gown might be worn for that procedure as a standard operating procedure (SOP) for all patients. Any additional barriers should be procedure-oriented (Standard Precautions) and used with the appropriate procedure each and every time.

Personal Hygiene

Proper personal hygiene is necessary before putting on PPE. Hair and fingernails harbor high levels of microorganisms and both should be thoroughly cleaned on a regular basis. As a general rule, hair should be pulled back from the face and pinned, and not hang on either side of the face or neck. Mustaches and beards must be neatly trimmed so that they can be covered by a mask and/or face shield. Rings or other hand jewelry, long nails and nail jewelry can cause difficulty in donning gloves, can interfere with your ability to wear the correct sized gloves, and can cause gloves to tear more easily. Long and artificial nails are often difficult to keep clean and have been linked to outbreaks of fungal and bacterial infections. Artificial nails should not be worn by DHCP.

The preferred method for hand hygiene depends on the type of procedure, the degree of contamination, and the desired persistence of antimicrobial action on the skin (see table below). For routine dental examinations and nonsurgical procedures, handwashing and hand antisepsis is achieved by using either a plain or antimicrobial soap and water. If the hands are not visibly soiled, an alcohol-based hand rub is adequate.

Tips & Hints

Handwashing is a cleaning process. Handwashing with water, or liquid detergent and water, is far better than not washing at all. The following criteria should be considered in selecting an appropriate handwash for your clinical setting:

1 · **Liquid handwash for routine handwashing**

2 · **An antimicrobial agent with a residual affect (substantivity) when indicated**

3 · **The use of a foot pump or electronic sensor for dispensing**
This helps to reduce contamination

4 · **Employee preferences, allergies, or sensitivities**

4 · **Cost comparison of equally effective and preferable products**

Hand Hygiene Methods and Indications

Method	Agent	Purpose	Duration (minimum)	Indication
Routine handwash	Water and nonantimicrobial soap (e.g., plain soap ɸ)	Remove soil and transient microorganisms	15 seconds§	Before and after treating each patient (e.g., before glove placement and after glove removal). After barehanded touching of inanimate objects likely to be contaminated by blood or saliva. Before leaving the dental operatory or the dental laboratory. When visibly soiled ⊖ Before regloving after removing gloves that are torn, cut, or punctured,
Antiseptic handwash	Water and antimicrobial soap (e.g., chlorhexidine, iodine and iodophors, chloroxylenol [PCIVIX], triclosan)	Remove or destroy transient microorganisms and reduce resident flora	15 seconds§	
Antiseptic hand rub	Alcohol-based hand rub ⊖	Remove or destroy transient microorganisms and reduce resident flora	Rub hands until the agent is dry ⊖	
Surgical antisepsis	Water and antimicrobial soap (e.g., chlorhexidine, iodine and iodophors, chloroxylenol [PCIVIX], triclosan) Water and non-antimicrobial soap (e.g., plain soap ɸ) followed by an alcohol-based surgical hand-scrub product with persistent activity	Remove or destroy transient microorganisms and reduce resident flora (persistent effect)	2-6 minutes Follow manufacturer instructions for surgical hand-scrub product with persistent activity ⊖**	Before donning sterile surgeon's gloves for surgical procedures ɸɸ

ɸ Pathogenic organisms have been found on or around bar soap during and after use (139). Use of liquid soap with hands-free dispensing controls is preferable.

§ Time reported as effective in removing most transient flora from the skin. For most procedures, a vigorous rubbing together of all surfaces of premoistened lathered hands and fingers for >15 seconds, followed by rinsing under a stream of cool or tepid water is recommended (9,120,123,140,141). Hands should always be dried thoroughly before donning gloves.

⊖ Alcohol-based hand rubs should contain 60%-95% ethanol or isopropanol and should not be used in the presence of visible soil or organic material. If using an alcohol-based hand rub, apply adequate amount to palm of one hand and rub hands together, covering all surfaces of the hands and fingers, until hands are dry. Follow manufacturer's recommendations regarding the volume of product to use. If hands feel dry after rubbing them together for 10-15 seconds, an insufficient volume of product likely was applied. The drying effect of alcohol can be reduced or eliminated by adding 1%-3% glycerol or other skin-conditioning agents (123).

**After application of alcohol-based surgical hand-scrub product with persistent activity as recommended, allow hands and forearms to dry thoroughly and immediately don sterile surgeon's gloves (144,145). Follow manufacturer instructions (122,123,137,146).

ɸɸ Before beginning surgical hand scrub, remove all arm jewelry and any hand jewelry that may make donning gloves more difficult, cause gloves to tear more readily (142,143), or interfere with glove usage (e.g., ability to wear the correct-sized glove or altered glove integrity).

Adapted from "Guidelines for Infection Control in Dental Health-Care Settings - 2003," MMWR, Dec. 19, 2003/Vol. 52/No. RR-17

Note: As of December 20, 2018 the FDA has indicated that the following ingredients in health care antiseptics are NOT generally recognized as safe and effective (chlorhexidine gluconate (CHG), iodine, iodophors, triclosan and some others). Any preparations with these ingredients cannot be legally sold unless they are the subject of an approved new drug application (NDA) or abbreviated NDA. Chloroxylenol (PCMX) and alcohol are OK for now and can be left in the table below. See: www.federalregister.gov/documents/2017/12/20/2017-27317/safety-and-effectiveness-of-health-care-antiseptics-topical-antimicrobial-drug-products-for

Suggested Handwashing Procedures

Routine Dental Procedures: Between patients and whenever donning or removing gloves, wash hands as follows. At the beginning of the day it may be necessary to complete 2 cycles of routine hand washing if the hands are visibly dirty following the initial routine handwashing.

1 · Wet hands, apply liquid soap with lukewarm water, avoid hot water.

2 · Rub hands together for at least 15 seconds; cover all surfaces of fingers, hands, and wrists.

3 · Interlace fingers and rub to cover all sides.

4 · Rinse under running water; dry thoroughly with disposable towels.

5 · If the faucet does not turn off automatically or have a foot-control, turn off faucet with the towel.

Antiseptic Hand Rub: Between patients if hands are clean and not contaminated.

1 · Decontaminate hands with an alcohol-based hand rub.

2 · Apply the product (follow manufacturer's directions for the amount to use) to the palm of one hand, and rub hands together.

3 · Rub hands vigorously, covering all surfaces of fingers and hands, until the hands are dry.

Oral Surgical Procedures: All clinical personnel who perform and assist in oral surgical procedures should perform hand antisepsis. This is accomplished by using either:

· water and an antimicrobial soap (i.e., an FDA-cleared antiseptic agent) or

· a non-antimicrobial soap (e.g., liquid, flake or foam plain soap) followed by an alcohol-based surgical hand-scrub product with persistent activity.

There are a variety of "best practice" techniques for surgical hand scrub. The specific dental healthcare practice setting should provide policies and procedures including education and training for surgical hand scrub. The specific technique to be used should be posted where the surgical scrub is to be performed as a continued reminder. The following is an example of a timed five-minute surgical hand scrub technique:

· Remove all jewelry (rings, watches, bracelets).

· Wash hands and arms with an antiseptic soap. Excessively hot water is harder on the skin, dries the skin, and is too uncomfortable to wash with for the recommended amount of time. However, because cold water prevents soap from lathering properly, soil and germs may not be washed away.

· Gently clean under the fingernail areas with a nail file or wooden nail stick to remove dirt and debris.

· Start timing. Scrub each side of each finger, between the fingers, and the back and front of the hand for a total of two minutes.

· Proceed to scrub the arms, keeping the hand higher than the arm at all times. This prevents bacteria-laden soap and water from contaminating the hand.

· Wash each side of the arm to three inches above the elbow for one minute.

· Repeat the process on the other hand and arm, keeping hands above elbows at all times. If the hand touches anything except the brush at any time, the scrub must be lengthened by one minute for the area that has been contaminated.

· Rinse hands and arms by passing them through the water in one direction only, from fingertips to elbow. Do not move the arm back and forth through the water.

· Proceed to the surgical treatment area holding hands above elbows.

· If the hands and arms are grossly soiled, the scrub time should be lengthened. However, vigorous scrubbing that causes the skin to become abraded should be avoided.

· At all times during the scrub procedure care should be taken not to splash water onto surgical attire.

· Once in the surgical treatment area, hands and arms should be dried using a sterile towel and aseptic technique. You are now ready to don your gown and sterile surgeon's gloves.

Other Suggestions:

The following are examples of additional concerns for hand hygiene.
Your Infection Control Coordinator may suggest or require others.

· The use of hand cream at the end of the day may reduce dryness that can occur from repeated handwashing and glove use. Dryness can cause microabrasions in your skin, making it more susceptible to exposure.

· Petroleum-based lotion formulations can weaken latex gloves and increase permeability. For that reason, lotions that contain petroleum or other oil emollients should only be used at the end of the work day.

· Store liquid hand-care products in either disposable closed containers or closed containers that can be washed and dried before refilling. Do not add soap or lotion to (i.e., top off) a partially empty dispenser.

· Store alcohol rubs away from heat sources (e.g., alcohol and gas torches, etc.).

Exposed areas of your body have the potential to be contaminated during a dental procedure. PPE is designed to protect your body and consists of clothing, barriers for the face and eyes, and gloves. We will discuss these in the manner you put them on, clothing first, followed by mask, eyewear and gloves. This order is also the reverse of what you change most often during the day, that is, you change gloves most often, masks less often, and clothing least of all.

Protective Clothing

When selecting protective clinic attire, it is important to select clothing that will be a barrier that is appropriate for the procedure being performed. While each dental office must determine what is appropriate attire for their specific procedures or office setting, keep in mind that protective clinic attire should be protective, sensible, comfortable and practical. In most cases, however, the extent of coverage of your protective clinic attire should be complete from the neck to the wrist, and at least to the bottom of the knees.

Clinical Clothing

Protective clinic attire must provide a barrier to any exposed skin and street clothes that have the potential to be contaminated during patient treatment or during other exposure-prone tasks such as operatory setup, take-down, instrument recirculation, laboratory activities, etc. Your employer or Coordinator must determine what attire is appropriate for your office. Additional barrier attire may be required for procedures that cause high levels of aerosolization or spatter.

Long-sleeved, high-collared laboratory coats that completely cover the torso may be the best barrier for exposed skin. Lab coats may also decrease the need for complete changes of street clothing at the end of the workday. Also, considering the amount of time DHCP spend sitting with knees on either side of a patient's head, it is likely that an area receiving a significant amount of foreign matter and splatter may be the thigh and knee area. For this reason, including reusable (washable) full-length pants as part of your protective attire might be appropriate if the lab coat doesn't cover the upper legs.

Note:

Protective clinical clothing is for clinical treatment areas only and should not be worn out of the office.

Laundering Clothing

Protective clinic attire should never be worn out of the office and should be changed at least daily, or more often if visually contaminated or wet and soaked through. After removal, it should be placed in labeled or color-coded containers for laundering. All protective clinic attire must be able to withstand repeated washing and heat drying. Silk and some acetate clothing will not stand up to the laundering cycle necessary for clinic attire. Cotton/polyester blends are more resistant to fluids than 100% cotton fabrics.

Standard precautions should be used in handling and laundering reusable protective clothing. Specific local regulations may apply. Employees cannot wash contaminated protective clinic attire at home. OSHA requires employers to be responsible for laundering of reusable protective clothing. When clothing is covered by protective clinical attire such as gowns or lab coats it is not expected to be contaminated with blood or other potentially infectious material. Therefore, uniforms or scrubs covered by protective clinical attire do not need to be handled as contaminated laundry and can be washed at home.

Disposable Clothing

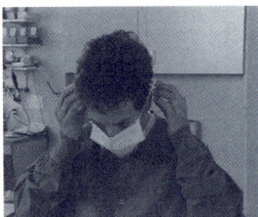

Disposable attire (as opposed to washable/reusable attire) is available from various distributors in the form of laboratory coats, bibs, aprons, etc. Attire must be replaced according to the manufacturer's directions, always changed when visibly soiled or penetrated with fluid, and should not be worn for more than one working day. This will vary with the types of exposures and the degree of contamination. After use, visibly soiled disposables may be considered as potentially infectious waste, and may be discarded with the general office trash, unless saturated with blood or saliva. The actual disposal is regulated by federal, state, or local waste regulations. When purchased in bulk and compared to the cost of laundry services or the installation and operation of an office washer and dryer, disposable attire may be a cost-effective alternative to washable dental clinic attire.

Other Suggestions:

Some dental procedures may require the use of additional PPE such as surgical booties or caps. This may apply for dental and surgical procedures that require sterile technique.

When increased aerosols are created during such procedures as ultrasonic scaling, extra attire barriers such as disposable aprons or gowns may be required. When other activities pose minimal risks of exposure, the barrier attire requirements may be modified for those tasks.

List the proper attire for your job:

_____

_____

⚠ Facial Barriers

It is important to barrier protect your face, nose and mouth from splash and spatter generated during dental treatment. The appropriate PPE includes face masks, protective eyewear and/or face shields.

Facemasks

A facemask provides barrier protection for the mucous membranes of the mouth and nose. The mask is an effective barrier until it becomes wet. The porosity of masks changes when soaked with moisture, reducing their filtration ability. Wet masks may "wick" or draw moisture to them. Masks should be disposed of when they become wet, or otherwise compromised by aerosols, spatter, or the healthcare worker's own breath. Masks should be removed before leaving the clinical area or office, and for contamination reasons, should not be worn resting against your neck or up on your head or hair, or carried by hand.

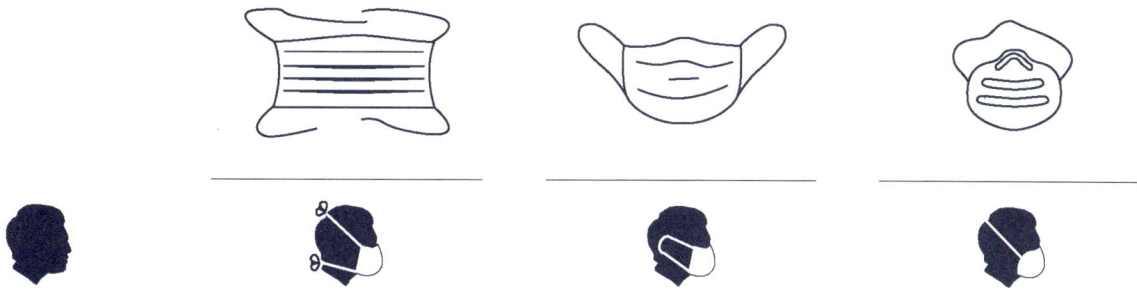

Q & A

Question: *How often do I change my mask?*

Answer: Changing masks between patients is recommended when procedures generate aerosols or the mask is damp from breath. Masks must always be changed when wet or compromised. There are no specific recommended time frames for mask changing, however by using logic in considering such factors as procedures performed, exposures to aerosols, saturation, and total time of use, you may then judge when a mask needs to be changed.

Masks come in many shapes and sizes; however, the two major styles are the molded dome mask and the flat pleated mask. Either style is appropriate as long as the mask fits the face and can be worn in such a way as to create a light seal over the nose and mouth. Most medical masks have a filtration effectiveness of 95-99% of 3-5 micron particles, as this will filter most particles encountered.

ASTM International (formerly known as the American Society for Testing and Materials) has designated three levels of fluid resistance of masks. The levels depend upon the amount of fluid and/or aerosols to which the masks will be exposed.

Question: *Where do I put my mask if I have to leave the room but will be returning to the patient in a few minutes?*

Answer: After removing your gloves and washing your hands, grasp the headstrap of your mask or the earloop (depending on the type of mask), remove it by the strap (not the mask itself), and place the mask on a disposable paper towel in the patient's operatory area. When returning, use the strap or ear loop to put the mask back on. Throw away the paper towel, wash your hands, and put on new gloves.

Protective Eyewear

Protect eyes from aerosols, splatter, debris and chemicals that may cause injury or infection. Choose protective eyewear made of high-impact plastic that covers the entire eye area from the eyebrow to the cheekbone, and on each side of the face. This includes solid (not vented) side shields. Prescription glasses used for eye protection must be equipped with solid side shields.

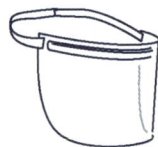

* Side Shields should be solid rather than slip-on or vented, as the latter do not provide protection against all exposures.

Tip

- For air abrasion or air polishing, use disposable shields to protect more expensive eyewear

Q & A

Question: *How do I clean my eyewear as it becomes contaminated during the course of the day?*

Answer: Clean with soap and water, or if visibly soiled, clean and disinfect reusable facial protective equipment (e.g., clinician and patient protective eyewear or face shields) between patients. When disinfectants are used, thoroughly rinse eyewear prior to use. Follow the eyewear manufacturer instructions for cleaning and de-contamination.

Question: *What if I wear prescription eyewear? I find it uncomfortable and distracting to wear safety glasses or goggles over my glasses.*

Answer: When choosing frames for prescription lenses, ensure that they adequately cover the entire eye area, and include straight temples with impact-resistant side coverage. Most opticians and dental equipment distributors carry prescription lenses in safety frames, as well as solid-side shield adaptors that attach to your eyewear. You can wear your own glasses provided they meet the standards for safety glasses.

Face Shields

For certain dental procedures, and at the discretion of the clinician, a full-face plastic shield may be appropriate. Procedures such as ultrasonic scaling, air polishing, and use of high-speed handpieces may generate large volumes of spatter and aerosol and can quickly saturate a mask. In these cases, the chin-length face shield may provide a longer lasting, more complete, barrier.

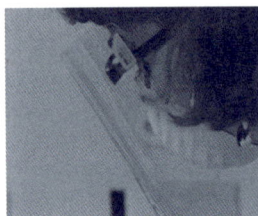

The size, design and materials of the face shield determine if there is a need to wear protective eyewear and/or a mask under the face shield. To provide better face and eye protection from splashes and sprays, a face shield should have crown and chin protection and wrap around the face to the point of the ear, which reduces the likelihood that a splash could go around the edge of the shield (worn in addition to a mask) and reach the eyes, nose or mouth.

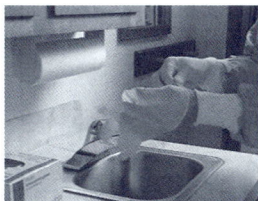

If the face shield is made of high impact plastic and is large enough to provide a protective barrier for the eyes, the face shield can be worn alone without protective eyewear. Disposable face shields designed for medical/dental personnel made of lightweight films that are attached to a surgical mask or fit loosely around the face should not be relied upon as optimal protection.

Face shields should be single-use, disposable, or, a reusable type that must be thoroughly decontaminated (i.e., cleaned and disinfected) between patients.

Gloves: Hand Barriers

Gloves should be worn whenever there is the potential for contact with blood, saliva, mucous membranes, hazardous or infections wastes, or chemical agents. Clinical treatment gloves are single-use items and *must be changed between each patient*. Gloves must be removed after patient treatment and before leaving the treatment area. In addition, torn or damaged gloves must be changed immediately. Handwashing must precede gloving and immediately follow glove removal.

Glove Types and Indications

Glove	Indication	Comment	Commercially available glove materials*	
			Material	Attributes**
Patient examination gloves §	Patient care, examinations, other nonsurgical procedures involving contact with mucous membranes, and laboratory procedures	Medical device regulated by the Food and Drug Administration (FDA). Nonsterile and sterile single-use disposable. Use for one patient and discard appropriately.	Natural-rubber latex (NRL) Nitrile Nitrile and chloroprene (neoprene) blends Nitrile & NRL blends Butadiene methyl methacrylate Polyvinyl chloride (PVC, vinyl) Polyurethane Styrene-based copolymer	1,2 2,3 2,3 1,2,3 2,3 4 4 4,5
Surgeon's gloves §	Surgical procedures	Medical device regulated by the FDA. Sterile and single-use disposable. Use for one patient and discard appropriately.	NRL Nitrile Chloroprene (neoprene) NRL and nitrile or chloroprene blends Synthetic polyisoprene Styrene-based copolymer Polyurethane	1,2 2, 3 2, 3 2, 3 2 4, 5 4
Nonmedical gloves	Housekeeping procedures (e.g., cleaning and disinfection) Handling contaminated sharps or chemicals Not for use during patient care	Not a medical device regulated by the FDA. Commonly referred to as utility, industrial, or general purpose gloves. Should be puncture- or chemical-resistant, depending on the task. Latex gloves do not provide adequate chemical protection. Sanitize after use.	NRL and nitrile or chloroprene blends Chloroprene (neoprene) Nitrile Butyl rubber Fluoroelastomer Polyethylene and ethylene vinyl alcohol copolymer	2,3 2, 3 2, 3 2, 3 3,4,6 3,4,6

* Physical properties can vary by material, manufacturer, and protein and chemical composition.
** Attributes
1 contains allergenic NRL proteins.
2 vulcanized rubber, contains allergenic rubber processing chemicals.
3 likely to have enhanced chemical or puncture resistance.
4 nonvulcanized and does not contain rubber processing chemicals.
5 inappropriate for use with methacrylates.
6 resistant to most methacrylates.
§ Medical or dental gloves include patient-examination gloves and surgeon's (i.e., surgical) gloves and are medical devices regulated by the FDA.
Only FDA-cleared medical or dental patient-examination gloves and surgical gloves can be used for patient care.

Adapted from "Guidelines for Infection Control in Dental Health-Care Settings - 2003," MMWR,Dec. 19, 2003/Vol. 52/No. RR-17

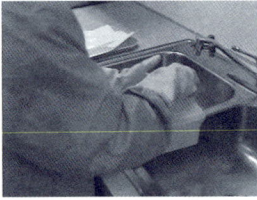

Before each procedure or task:

1 · Wash and dry hands thoroughly (see Handwashing Protocol, pg. 3-5).

2 · Put on fresh gloves: Appropriate for the procedure/task to be performed.

3 · After completion of procedure or task, remove gloves and then wash and dry hands, or use alcohol rub according to the Handwashing Protocol. Never reglove without performing hand hygiene.

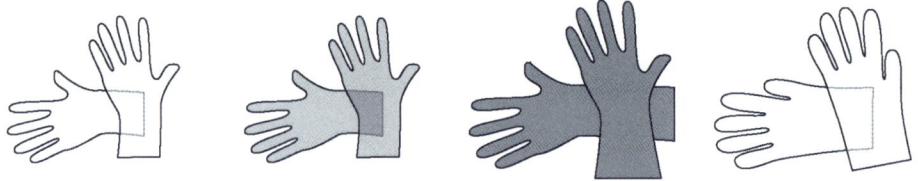

The Right Glove for Each Task

There are several types of gloves on the market, and in the course of your job, you may use different gloves for different tasks. Use the table "Glove Types and Indications" and the recommendations below to select the proper glove.

• Wear clinical gloves when a potential exists for contacting blood, saliva, other potentially infectious materials (OPIM), or mucous membranes.

• Wear a new pair of clinical gloves for each patient, remove them promptly after use and either wash hands or use an alcohol hand rub to avoid transfer of microorganisms to other patients or environments.

• Remove gloves that are torn, cut, or punctured as soon as feasible and wash hands before putting on a new pair of gloves.

• Do not wash surgeon's or patient examination gloves before use or wash, disinfect, or sterilize gloves for reuse.

• Ensure that appropriate gloves in the correct size are readily accessible.

• Use appropriate gloves (e.g., puncture-and chemical-resistant utility gloves) when cleaning instruments and performing housekeeping tasks involving contact with blood or OPIM.

• Consult with glove manufacturers regarding the chemical compatibility of glove material and dental materials used.

Sterile Surgeon's Gloves and Double Gloving During Oral Surgical Procedures

• Wear sterile surgeon's gloves when performing oral surgical procedures.

• No recommendation is offered regarding the effectiveness of wearing two pairs of gloves to prevent disease transmission during oral surgical procedures. The majority of studies among HCP and DHCP have demonstrated a lower frequency of inner glove perforation and visible blood on the surgeon's hands when double gloves are worn; however, the effectiveness of wearing two pairs of gloves in preventing disease transmission has not been demonstrated.

Tips & Hints

- Refer to the manufacturer's instructions for the shelf life and storage requirements of latex gloves. For example, gloves can be affected by temperature, humidity, and light. They should be stored in a dark constant environment of moderate temperature and low humidity.

- The U.S. Food and Drug Administration (FDA) has banned the sale of powdered gloves. Some individuals have a sensitivity to the powders used inside some gloves and/or they may be allergic to latex proteins that leach from powdered latex gloves and adhere to the powder. The residual powder from the glove is easily spread to clothing and into the air and may pose a risk of a respiratory reaction in allergic individuals (patients and workers).

Gloves are available in many sizes. They are also available in right, left, or ambidextrous and should fit snugly but comfortably on the hand without being tight. Gloves that do not fit appropriately can increase fatigue and potentially lead to muscle and nerve injury.

Q & A

Question: *How do I dispose of my gloves after use?*

Answer: In most circumstances, gloves can be thrown away with general waste. However, this may be dependent upon local and state medical waste regulations. See Course #9.

Contact Dermatitis and Latex Hypersensitivity

Occupationally related contact dermatitis can develop from frequent and repeated use of hand hygiene products, exposure to chemicals, and glove use. Contact dermatitis is classified as either irritant or allergic. Irritant contact dermatitis is common, nonallergic, and develops as dry, itchy, irritated areas on the skin around the area of contact. By comparison, allergic contact dermatitis (type IV hypersensitivity) can result from exposure to accelerators and other chemicals used in the manufacture of rubber gloves (e.g., natural rubber latex, nitrile, and neoprene), as well as from other chemicals found in the dental practice setting (e.g., methacrylates and glutaraldehyde). Allergic contact dermatitis often manifests as a rash beginning hours after contact and, similar to irritant dermatitis, is usually confined to the area of contact.

Types of Reaction	Symptoms/Signs	Cause	Prevention/Management
(1) Irritant Contact Dermatitis	Itchy, red, inflamed, scaling, dry and cracked skin	Direct skin irritation by gloves, powder, soaps/detergents, incomplete hand drying	Obtain medical diagnosis, dermatology consultation, avoid irritant product, assure glove material provides proper barrier; consider alternative gloves/products, cotton/liners
(2) Allergic Contact Dermatitis (Type IV delayed hypersensitivity or allergic contact sensitivity)	Itchy, red, inflamed, scaling, dry and cracked blistering (similar to poison ivy reaction); 24-72 hrs. after contact	Accelerators (e.g. thiurams, carbamates, benzothiazoles) processing chemicals (e.g., biocides, antioxidants) NRL Consider penetration of glove barrier by chemicals	Obtain medical diagnosis, dermatology consultation; identify chemical. Consider use of glove liners such as cotton. Use alternative glove material without chemical. Assure glove material is suitable for intended use (proper barrier)
(3) NRL Allergy - IgE mediated (Type 1 immediate hypersensitivity)		NRL proteins; direct contact/breathing NRL proteins including glove powder containing NRL proteins, from powdered NRL gloves/environment	For (3)(a), (3)(b), and (3)(c): Obtain medical diagnosis, allergy consultation; substitute non-NRL gloves and other non-NRL products for affected worker Eliminate exposure to glove powder - use of reduced allergen, powder free gloves or non-NRL gloves for coworkers (assure glove material provides a proper barrier) Clean NRL-containing powder from environment Consider NRL safe environment
(3)(a) Localized contact urticaria	Hives in area of contact with NRL	Wearing NRL gloves or other direct contact with NRL allergenic proteins	
(3)(b) Other Allergic Manifestation	Allergic rhinitis, allergic conjunctivitis, asthma	Exposure to aerosolized NRL allergenic protein. Key role - glove powder	
(3)(c) Generalized Reaction	Manifesting as: generalized urticaria, asthma, upper respiratory symptoms, and/or flushing, rapid pulse, falling blood pressure, weakness. Can progress to anaphylactic shock	Exposure to NRL allergenic proteins by any one of several routes	

Reference: OSHA SHIB 01-28-2008, Potential for Allergy to Natural Rubber Latex Gloves and other Natural Rubber Products; http://www.osha.gov/dts/shib/shib012808.html

Latex allergy (type I hypersensitivity to latex proteins) can be a more serious systemic allergic reaction, usually beginning within minutes of exposure but sometimes occurring hours later and producing varied symptoms. More common reactions include runny nose, sneezing, itchy eyes, scratchy throat, hives, and itchy burning skin sensations. More severe symptoms include asthma marked by difficult breathing, coughing spells, and wheezing; cardiovascular and gastrointestinal ailments; and in rare cases, anaphylaxis and death.

Natural rubber latex proteins responsible for latex allergy are attached to glove powder. When powdered latex gloves are worn, more latex protein reaches the skin. In addition, when powdered latex gloves are donned or removed, latex protein/powder particles become aerosolized and can be inhaled, contacting mucous membranes. As a result, allergic patients and DHCP can experience cutaneous, respiratory, and conjunctical symptoms related to latex protein exposure.

How Large a Problem is Latex Allergies?

The American Dental Association (ADA) began investigating the prevalence of type I latex hypersensitivity among DHCP at the ADA annual meeting in 1994. In 1994 and 1995, approximately 2,000 dentists, hygienists, and assistants volunteered for skin-prick testing. Data demonstrated that 6.2% of those tested were positive for type I latex hypersensitivity. Data from the subsequent five years of this ongoing cross-sectional study indicated a decline in prevalence from 8.5% to 4.3%. This downward trend is similar to that reported by other studies and might be related to use of latex gloves with lower allergen content.

- Educate DHCP regarding the signs, symptoms, and diagnoses of skin reactions associated with frequent hand hygiene and glove use. Encourage testing if allergy is suspected.
- Discuss latex allergy with all patients and refer for medical consultation if latex allergy is suspected.
- Ensure a latex-safe or latex-free environment where indicated.
- Have latex alternatives available, such as gloves and other devices.
- Have emergency treatment kits with latex-free products available at all times.

How can Latex Allergy be Prevented?

- Appropriate barrier protection is necessary when handling infectious materials. When choosing latex gloves, use powder-free gloves with reduced protein content.

- If you are going to use latex gloves, limit their use to clinical intra-oral procedures.

- Do not use oil-based hand creams or lotions with latex gloves unless they have been shown to reduce latex-related problems.

- After removing latex gloves, wash hands with a mild soap and dry thoroughly or use an alcohol-based hand rub.

- Ensure that DHCP use good housekeeping practices to remove latex-containing dust from the workplace. Ventilation filters and vacuum bags need to be changed regularly.

- Screen high-risk DHCP for latex allergy symptoms periodically and evaluate current prevention strategies whenever a DHCP is diagnosed with latex allergy.

- If you develop symptoms of latex allergy, avoid direct contact with gloves and other latex containing products until you can see a physician experienced in diagnosing and treating latex allergy.

- Check label for additional information.

The Right Glove for You

In addition to being the appropriate size, gloves must not be irritating to your skin. Some individuals may have sensitivities or even allergies to chemicals used in glove manufacturing, or to the naturally occurring latex proteins in latex gloves. Reactions may range from irritant contact dermatitis to an actual allergic response. Not all reactions are due to latex exposure. It is important to have any reaction definitively diagnosed by a qualified physician, such as an allergist.

Other dental products such as dental dams and straps on face masks, may also contain latex. It is important to identify all latex-containing products so they can be replaced with non-latex containing-materials or avoided when a patient or employee is truly latex allergic.

If you have a reaction to the gloves you should:

1 · Notify your Infection Control Coordinator or Employer.

2 · Determine if you are performing proper handcare.

3 · Determine if the reaction is to the hand hygiene agent (ex. soap), powder, and/or other glove material.

4 · Have a definitive diagnosis by an allergist in order to determine the appropriate accommodations in the workplace.

5 · If you are allergic to certain gloves, select an appropriate and compatible alternative glove. Ask your Infection Control Coordinator for assistance.

6 · Report any adverse reactions to the FDA.

List four different types of gloves and an example for a procedure where it is used:

1._____

2._____

3._____

4._____

Discussion

Below are some questions that will assist you in a discussion with your Infection Control Coordinator or Safety Officer.

You have now completed the workbook segment for Course #3. Below are three sample questions that will also assist you in your discussion with your Infection Control Coordinator, employer, or dentist, and other staff members..

Question: *I've had problems with my face mask. Every day, in the late afternoon, my face begins to itch and there is a red rash around where the mask was. What should I do?*

Answer: First, speak with your Infection Control Coordinator about trying a mask made from different material. If, after switching, the rash continues, try seeing a dermatologist to isolate the exact irritant.

Question: *I treat a lot of very young patients, including my five-year-old nephew, and a lot of them are frightened by all the personal protective equipment I wear. Can I take any of it off while treating them?*

Answer: It is important to follow Standard Precautions at all times for all patients to protect not only yourself, but all of your patients. This means that you must consider every child, no matter how small, potentially infectious. This includes family members. Why risk passing a cold or flu from one patient to another, regardless of who they are?

There are things you can do to help young children relax: The first and most important is to talk to them, explaining 'why' you're doing 'what' you're doing. Let them ask questions and answer them honestly. This short face-to-face time also allows them to see and trust you before you put on your PPE. Wear colorful masks or draw animals, flowers, or designs on plain ones. You could also let young patients draw or put stickers on your mask before you put it on, or let them take a mask that they colored home. If you have a particularly anxious child in the chair, you might let him/her play with a blown-up rubber glove (if they are not allergic) which can be held during treatment.

Question: *My hands are breaking out from the gloves I'm wearing. What can I do?*

Answer: First, evaluate your handcare procedures. Are you fully drying your hands after each washing? Have you taken off all your jewelry? Are you using lukewarm, not hot, water to wash your hands? (See page 3-7.) Should you discontinue or begin using a hand cream? If you are wearing a powdered glove, switch to a glove without powder. If the problem does not clear up, try a different type or brand of gloves. You should also seek an allergist's opinion.

Objectives

Upon completion of this course on a practical program for exposure control, you will be able to:

1. Explain the role of Standard Operating Procedures (SOPs) in exposure control.

2. Explain the role of assessment in the development of effective SOPs.

3. Assess the infection control needs of the operatory setting in a dental office.

4. Explain the process of operatory turnaround, also called operatory processing.

5. Differentiate between a cleaner and disinfectant.

6. Differentiate between disinfection and environmental surface barrier protection.

7. Identify three methods of reducing contaminated aerosols in the operatory.

8. Explain how contaminated sharps are isolated in the practice setting.

9. Identify specific infection control considerations unique to digital radiology.

10. Identify specific infection control considerations unique to the dental laboratory setting.

Focus

With all the factors affecting dentistry, the best way to practice safe dentistry is to take a logical approach to your day, integrating many factors: the science of infection control, OSHA regulations, recommendations from the CDC, and from the various professional organizations, and the desire for efficiency in your dental practice.

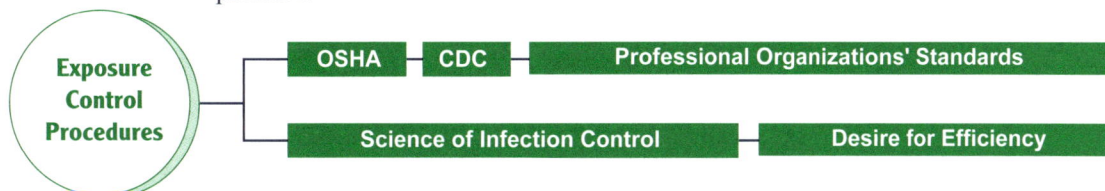

Exposure Control Procedures

OSHA — **CDC** — **Professional Organizations' Standards**

Science of Infection Control — **Desire for Efficiency**

First Steps

An initial step in developing an Exposure Control Program is to assess the infection control and safety needs of the practice. One way is for the Infection Control Coordinator and/or employer to walk through the operatories, laboratory, radiology processing area, and instrument reprocessing area observing how tasks are currently performed and identifying associated risks or hazards.

Questions you may need to answer include:

- **Which procedures do you perform that involve potential hazards?**
- **Are these hazards physical, chemical, or infectious?**
- **How can these hazards be reduced?**

List the step-by-step process of completing a given task by combining all of the factors listed above that affect your workday, providing a realistic picture of what is required of you in your practice. This list can then be used to develop detailed instructions for performing various tasks in the practice. These are called Standard Operating Procedures (SOPs) and are the foundation of your Exposure Control Program. The goals of developing SOPs include:

- Developing a standard set of procedures to guide the dental team when performing tasks.

- Reducing the risk of occupational exposure incidents.

- Establishing consistent methods of compliance with regulations and recommendations.

- Establishing a culture of safety for personnel and patients.

SOP's and Methods of Compliance

We use the SOP to designate the written plans required for your office. Your practice, however, may be using another term, such as Methods of Compliance. Regardless of the name used, these plans should be located in your practice's compliance plan, which we refer to as the Infection Control/Exposure Control Plan. Be aware that you may have to locate the SOP for a particular procedure to help understand how this course relates to your practice.

Notes:

This course uses "operatory preparation" and "turnaround" to demonstrate how to develop safe and efficient office exposure control procedures. We also use the term "operatory processing" as we discuss a systematic approach to operatory turnaround.

Several times during this and other courses, you should refer to your Infection Control/Exposure Control Plan to locate the SOP relating to the topic of discussion. If your practice uses other terms for the Infection Control/Exposure Control Plan or Standard Operating Procedures, use the corresponding written plans.

Your Role in Safety

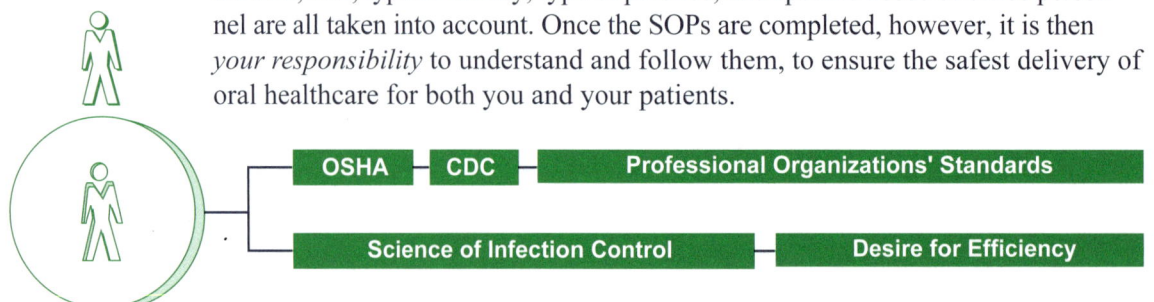

If all of your practice's SOPs are written, what is your role? In developing SOPs, the task, risk, type of facility, type of practice, and specific needs of office personnel are all taken into account. Once the SOPs are completed, however, it is then *your responsibility* to understand and follow them, to ensure the safest delivery of oral healthcare for both you and your patients.

OSHA — CDC — Professional Organizations' Standards

Science of Infection Control — Desire for Efficiency

In addition to following an SOP, you play a *critical* role in evaluating and updating SOPs. You must use your personal expertise to continually reevaluate SOPs for the tasks you perform, which will help you to work safely and efficiently.

Assessment

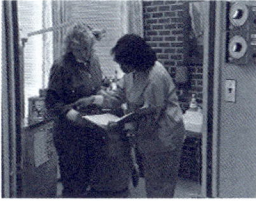

Take a minute to think about, look at, and then assess the operatory in which you work. Although you can't totally eliminate hazards, there are steps you can take to promote a healthy and safe environment. Is the area clean? Are the counters cluttered with any unnecessary supplies? Are any storage or supply containers open? Are patient records or papers in an area of exposure?

The goal of this assessment is to make your operatory as simple to clean and prepare as possible. If the operatory contains unnecessary items, consider moving them to a storage area. Your Infection Control Coordinator can work with you to streamline the operatory and thereby begin to maximize efficiency.

List a few non-essential items in your operatory that could be removed to facilitate easier cleaning.

_____

_____

_____

_____

_____

Time Management

Once you have streamlined your operatories and have taken exposure control factors into account, you are ready to evaluate each step of the Operatory Processing SOP to determine a realistic time frame in which to effectively complete this procedure. This process, and the use of its results, is called "time management" and allows you to schedule appointments with enough time and staff support to accomplish each task. With proper time management, you need not feel rushed between patients.

Tips & Hints

After an SOP is developed in your practice, and staff have had an opportunity to be trained for the procedure, monitor their efforts using a stopwatch (time-motion assessment). This will produce realistic time frames for completing each given procedure and may even show areas that can be modified for improved efficiency. Keep in mind your goal is to streamline your tasks and find realistic time frames to aid in scheduling, not to turn operatory processing or any procedure into a race.

Note:

This course concentrates on operatory preparation and turnaround as an example of environmental exposure control. Before incorporating this information directly into your own daily routine you should consider:

- **Office design and organization**
- **The number of clinical staff members**
- **The number and types of tasks to be performed**
- **SOPs for completing these tasks**
- **State and Local regulations**
- **Recommendations from the CDC**
- **Regulations from OSHA**

Terminology

Before we begin, let's review some basic terminology:

- Bioburden: Amount of biological or organic material, such as blood and saliva, on a surface.

- Cleaning: to remove visible debris and dirt by use of a detergent and mechanical means prior to disinfection and/or barrier protection.

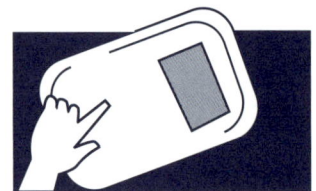

- Clinical Contact Surfaces: Surfaces that are touched by contaminated hands, instruments, devices, or other items, while providing dental or medical care, or while performing activities that support dental or medical care.

- Disinfection: The process of decontamination, which kills most microorganisms, with the exception of spore-forming organisms left on a surface after cleaning.

- Disinfectant: Used on hard inanimate surfaces and objects to destroy or irreversibly inactivate infectious fungi, viruses, and bacteria, but not necessarily bacterial endospores. Disinfectants are further discussed in Course #6.

- EPA-Registered Disinfectant: EPA registers three types of disinfectants based on data submitted by the manufacturer: Limited, General (or Broad-spectrum), and Hospital.

- EPA-Registered Hospital Disinfectant: a general or broad-spectrum disinfectant that is also effective against certain bacteria. These disinfectants are among the most critical to infection control and are used on medical and dental equipment, floors, walls, bed linens, toilet seats, and other surfaces.

- Housekeeping Surfaces: Environmental surfaces that are not involved in the direct delivery of dental care (for example, floors, or walls).

- Microbial Dose Load: The dose load of microorganisms present in a specific area.

- Noncritical Surfaces: An item or surface in the treatment area that does not touch or penetrate human tissue, but may become contaminated by aerosolization, spatter, or contact with contaminated items.

The Initial Preparation of an Operatory Involves Three Basic Steps:

1. Clean and Disinfect   **2. Barrier Protect**   **3. Plan Treatment**

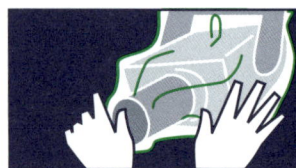

These steps are logical, in both their importance and the order in which you perform them. It is your responsibility to take the theory and the SOPs for office preparation, and combine them with a time management approach, in order to maximize efficiency.

Step 1: Clean and Disinfect

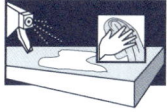

To ensure a clean operatory, all surfaces and equipment that have the potential to become contaminated from hand contact, aerosols, spatter, or other contaminated items must be cleaned. Cleaning is necessary *prior* to disinfection or the initial placement of barriers. If a clinical contact surface cannot be cleaned, disinfectants will not work and barriers must be used.

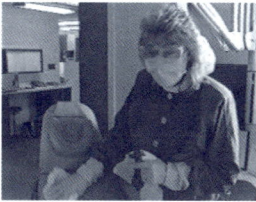

As you look around the operatory, how do you decide what needs to be cleaned? You should consult the SOP for Operatory Processing in your practice's Infection Control/Exposure Control Plan for a specific list of items and surfaces in your operatory that are either cleaned and then disinfected, or that are cleaned and then barrier protected. These noncritical items and surfaces include countertops and other surfaces, supply cabinets, containers, operatory chairs, and various dental equipment and supplies that are at risk for contamination but that are not used intraorally.

The goal of cleaning is to decrease the number of microorganisms present to reduce bioburden. Once the bioburden is decreased, disinfection is more effective. In other words, you want to clean the dirt off the surface first, to allow the chemical to make contact and then disinfect the surface.

Cleaning

Cleaning can be done with anything that is a cleansing agent, such as water and detergent. The higher the detergent or "surfactant" quality of the agent, the better it is at breaking up dirt and debris. Water is *required* to enhance the cleaning process.

Tips & Hints

- **In an effort to save time, you may want to use one product in two steps to clean and disinfect the operatory. A disinfectant that is also a good cleaner must contain a surfactant. These products, which will be covered in greater detail in Course #6, are registered with the Environmental Protection Agency (EPA) and if the surface is contaminated with blood, the product must be labeled with the *Mycobacterium tuberculosis* kill claim on the outside of the product container.**

- **With all products, it is important to follow the manufacturer's instructions for use in handling and storage.**

- **Products that contain a surfactant will most likely state in the directions that the product can be used for both cleaning and disinfecting. Products without a surfactant will state that cleaning is necessary prior to the use of that particular disinfectant.**

No matter what products you use to clean and disinfect, all are intended for use on inanimate surfaces and not on human tissue. To protect yourself from a chemical exposure, use appropriate PPE, and follow all the barrier precautions listed on the product label or found on the product's Safety Data Sheet (SDS). PPE usually includes barrier attire, mask, eyewear, and gloves, such as heavy-duty utility or nitrile-rubber. Some disinfectants may require special ventilation.

Observe these steps when using one product to both clean and disinfect.

1. **Spray** the surface with a surfactant-containing hospital-level disinfectant with tuberculocidal activity.

2. **Wipe** the moist surface with toweling.

3. **Spray** the surface again, leaving the chemical on the surface for the designated time to achieve tuberculocidal kill, according to the manufacturer's instructions, usually letting it air dry.

If you choose to use different chemicals for cleaning and disinfecting, the process is almost the same: you spray the cleanser on the surface and wipe it off, then spray the disinfectant on the surface and leave it on the surface for the designated time to achieve tuberculocidal kill, according to the manufacturer's instructions.

An alternative is to use disinfectant wipes; however, they must be used according to the manufacturer's instructions.

What product(s) are used in your practice as cleaners and surface disinfectants?

_____
_____
_____

List the surfaces that are cleaned and disinfected in the operatory you normally reprocess.

_____
_____
_____
_____
_____
_____
_____

Step 2: Barrier Protection

Barriers are preferred over disinfectants because they reduce exposure to chemical germicides and save time in operatory processing. In addition, some items in the operatory cannot be effectively cleaned and disinfected. Those surfaces that have ridges, grooves, switches, electrical components, or attachments, are more effectively managed if they are barrier protected between patients. Barrier protection is the process of isolating surfaces with a covering; it is not a replacement for the cleaning process, but rather an alternative to the repeated cleaning and disinfection process. Saliva ejector holders, tray handles, light switches, light handles, the water syringe handle, and other frequently touched items should be considered for barrier protection. It may not be necessary to clean items that are barrier protected *between patients*, but at a minimum these items should be cleaned:

- **At the beginning of the day**
- **At the end of the day**
- **During the day, if the barriers are compromised and the surfaces under them become contaminated**

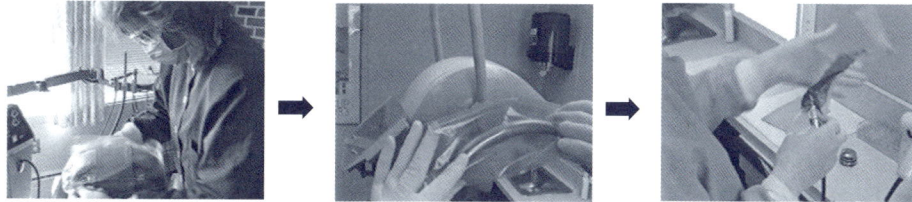

You may use more than one kind of barrier in the operatory, depending upon the item or surface to be protected. Barriers can be made of different materials but they must all be fluid-proof. Because it is easy to use, plastic is currently the most widely used form of barrier protection. If you use plastic wrap, it must meet the FDA weight standards for food wrap. This will be stated on the outside of the product container. Commercial medical surface covers and barriers are best to use.

Note:

The FDA considers barriers medical devices, if they are marketed as products to be used in the clinical areas. These barriers must go through the FDA and receive approval to market in this way. Other products, such as food wrap, if not marketed as medical devices, do not need to go through this process.

Barrier protection may also save time that would otherwise be used in the continual cleaning and disinfecting process. The time a chemical must remain on the surface to achieve the proper tuberculocidal kill is usually several minutes, thus, the use of barriers can significantly reduce this waiting time. In reality, you must assess your operatory and decide how best to save time, versus the cost of barriers or the ease of placing barriers. Through experimentation, you will find the right mix of barriers and cleaned and disinfected surfaces.

The SOP in your practice's Infection Control/Exposure Control Plan provides instructions for which equipment and surfaces in the operatory should be barrier protected.

Using your practice's SOP for Operatory Preparation, look at the number & types of barriers that you use.

List the items to be barrier-protected and what barriers to use in the operatory you normally reprocess.

_____

_____

_____

_____

_____

_____

Cleaning and disinfecting surfaces between patients

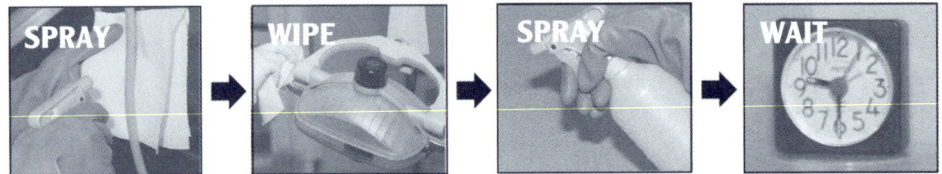

Covering surfaces with impermeable barriers

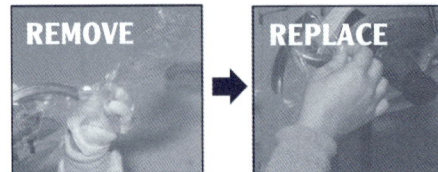

Note: When using surface barriers between patients, cleaning and disinfection are only necessary if a barrier has torn or been punctured, or if the surface beneath it has been otherwise contaminated.

Step 3: Plan Treatment

Anticipating the treatment needs of each patient, or planning patient treatment, is another method of promoting an efficient, safe working environment. Not only does it save time, but it also reduces the chance for contamination, since the number of items handled is minimized to only what is necessary for patient care.

Preview Record to Plan Treatment

To efficiently plan treatment, carefully review the patient's record and treatment plan. Then, select the types and amounts of supplies needed and keep in mind that unused items will have to be discarded or resterilized, if not used. This can be costly in terms of time and money.

Planning Involves:

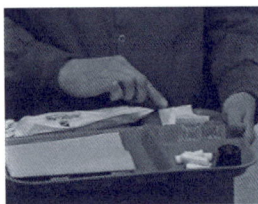

1. **Selecting the materials and supplies appropriate to the procedure**
   This includes, but is not limited to:
   - **Unit dosed disposable items, such as gauze, cotton rolls, and cotton pellets**
   - **Preparation of dental dam setup, if appropriate**
   - **Sterilized or new burs**
   - **Local anesthesia setup, including a sharps container and a safe needle recapping device**
   - **Treatment-specific dental materials**
2. **Preparing suitable patient barriers, including bib/drape, & protective eyewear**

Summary

Cleaning, disinfecting, barrier-protecting, and treatment planning are the major steps of operatory preparation. As you look back at the number of procedures to be performed, and the number of times you do them each day, the need for an organized operatory and time management is essential.

Research has shown that the small-bore plastic tubing used to provide coolant and irrigating water for dental procedures is frequently contaminated with large numbers of potentially pathogenic microorganisms. This phenomenon results from colonization of biofilms on water-bearing surfaces in the dental unit. Biofilms are slime-protected microbial communities attached to the inner surface of the tubing that may harbor bacteria, fungi, protozoans, and even microscopic nematode worms. The small interior diameter of the tubing greatly increases the surface area available for biofilm formation in comparison to the volume of water in the lines. The result is high concentrations of microorganisms in water delivered to the dental patient.

Although most of the organisms isolated by researchers are the same kinds of aquatic bacteria found in smaller numbers in drinking water, potentially pathogenic bacteria such as *Pseudomonas aeruginosa*, *Legionella* species and oral flora have been recovered. Since dental treatment water is often used for invasive procedures and may also be delivered in the form of droplets or aerosols, pathogenic organisms may enter a susceptible host via the gastrointestinal, respiratory, or circulatory system. Despite this potential hazard, there are very few documented cases of illness associated with exposure to contaminated dental treatment water. Nevertheless, therapeutic use of fluids that fail to meet accepted standards for drinking water is inconsistent with the basic principles of infection control.

Waterline Treatment

The CDC Guidelines for Infection Control in Dental Healthcare Settings - 2003 state that only sterile fluids should be used for procedures in which bone is exposed (this includes most periodontal and oral surgery procedures). No conventional dental unit can deliver irrigating solutions consistent with this guideline. In order to provide sterile solutions, a surgical device must use either a sterile disposable or sterilizable water delivery system. The use of a sterilizable bulb syringe or disposable irrigating syringe with sterile irrigating fluid offers the simplest acceptable approach.

Standards also exist for safe drinking water quality, as established by EPA, the American Public Health Association (APHA), and the American Water Works Association (AWWA); they have set limits for heterotrophic bacteria of ≤500 CFU/mL of drinking water. Thus, the number of bacteria in water used as a coolant/irrigant for nonsurgical dental procedures should be as low as reasonably achievable and, at a minimum, ≤500 CFU/mL, the regulatory standard for safe drinking water established by EPA and APHA/AWWA.

Note:

- A boil-water advisory is a public health announcement that occurs when the public water supply is contaminated, Specific and up-to-date recommendations for dental practice settings during a boil-water advisory are at cdc.gov/OralHealth/infection-control/factsheets/boilwater.htm.

Recommendations:

- Use water that meets EPA regulatory standards for drinking water (i.e., ≤500 CFU/mL of heterotrophic water bacteria) for routine dental treatment output water.
- Consult with the dental unit manufacturer for appropriate methods and equipment to maintain the recommended quality of dental water.
- Follow recommendations for monitoring water quality provided by the manufacturer of the unit or waterline treatment product or device.
- Discharge water and air for a minimum of 20–30 seconds after each patient, from any device connected to the dental water system that enters the patient's mouth (e.g., handpieces, ultrasonic scalers, and air/water syringes).
- Consult the dental unit manufacturer on the need for periodic maintenance of anti-retraction mechanisms.

Technologies and Guidance

Currently marketed technologies include independent water reservoirs, filtration, or various combinations as approaches to control, eliminate, or prevent biofilm formation in dental unit water lines.

The use of independent reservoirs without effective control or elimination of biofilms will not be effective, even if sterile water is used in the bottle. Care must be taken when handling independent reservoirs to avoid contaminating the water system with human skin or intestinal bacteria. The dental unit manufacturer should have a recommended waterline treatment regimen, which should be followed.

Dental Unit Water Quality: Organization for Safety, Asepsis and Prevention White Paper and Recommendations – 2018 published in the Journal of Dental Infection Control and Safety Volume 1/Issue 1, provides more detail on the background of dental unit water quality as well as recommendations. To read the full article, visit: osapjdics.scholasticahq.com

The CDC guideline further advises DHCWs to use and monitor the effectiveness of anti-retraction valves. Although many older dental units were equipped with active devices to prevent retraction of oral fluids, most contemporary systems are passively non-retracting. DHCWs should contact the unit manufacturer to determine whether to test or replace anti-retraction devices.

Chairside Exposure Control

Hazards can be reduced through a clean and organized operatory. What other ways exist to minimize the risks you face each day? An assessment of your work habits provides a number of clues for decreasing hazards during patient treatment, and may promote "chairside exposure control."

Chairside Exposure Control Focuses on:

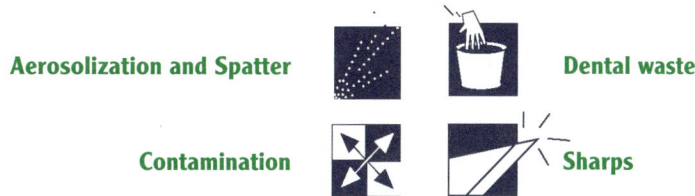

Aerosolization and Spatter

Dental waste

Contamination

Sharps

1. Reducing Aerosolization and Spatter

Each time you use an ultrasonic scaler, a high-speed handpiece, or an air/water syringe, aerosols and spatter are created, by diminishing aerosols and spatter, you reduce the risk of contamination or exposure. There are a number of simple ways to minimize or protect yourself from aerosols and spatter:

1. **Use high-volume evacuation (suction).** This limits the amount of aerosolized saliva.

2. **Use a dental dam whenever possible.** This reduces the amount of oral fluids contacted during a procedure containing them beneath the dam, and minimizes the chance that the patient will swallow materials.

3. **Use additional PPE barriers,** such as disposable gowns and face shields, as necessary. This is especially important when doing procedures that increase aerosolization, such as ultrasonic scaling and oral surgery procedures.

4. **Use a preprocedural mouthrinse for each patient.** There is no scientific evidence that the use of a preprocedural mouthrinse will reduce the risk of or prevent transmission of disease. This will also not directly reduce aerosolization, but it may reduce the microbial dose load generated in aerosols and spatter. Types of rinses include:

   • **First-generation antimicrobial mouthrinse, alcohol-based:** An over-the-counter mouthwash, with antiseptic agents, that can be used with any patient who can tolerate an alcohol-based rinse (short-term antimicrobial)

   • **First-generation antimicrobial mouthrinse, alcohol-free:** A mouth rinse, with antiseptic agents, for those patients with alcohol intolerance (short-term antimicrobial)

   • **Second-generation antimicrobial mouthrinses:** A prescription mouthwash for use during more invasive and aerosol-prone procedures. These are antiseptic agents, with substantivity. They have a wider range of antimicrobial kill and inactivation, and last longer (long-term antimicrobial)

   • **Water:** For mechanical reduction, which washes away contaminants

These practices may reduce the microbial dose load in the oral cavity.

Contamination often occurs without anyone noticing. During treatment, you may reach for an instrument that is stored in a cabinet, make notes in the patient's record, answer the phone, or adjust your glasses. These events, and others, can cause the potential transfer of microorganisms. Although there are two simple ways to reduce contamination, they are not always realistic or practical:

- **Don't interrupt treatment.**
- **Don't touch anything that is not essential for patient treatment.**

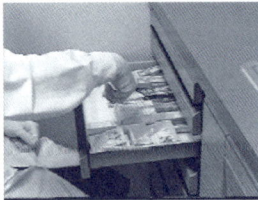

There will be times when treatment must be interrupted or when you will have to leave the operatory. If this happens, remove and dispose of your gloves, and perform hand hygiene (Course #3), so you don't contaminate items outside the operatory. If you need to leave the clinical area, follow the procedures covered in Course #3 for removing and protecting your face mask, and remember not to touch your eyewear with your bare hands. When you return, put on your mask, perform hand hygiene, put on new gloves, and resume treatment.

During treatment, avoid touching unprotected surfaces and equipment, including the patient's record. If you must enter drawers, cabinets, or containers once treatment begins, use forceps or overgloves to retrieve items. Forceps and overgloves are used for one patient only; forceps are sterilized after use and overgloves are disposed of as appropriate.

Taking Notes

While you may need to make chart entries while in the operatory, the patient's record poses a unique challenge because it's very difficult to decontaminate. Ideally, records should be left outside the treatment area, with notes made after treatment is completed. If the record must be kept in the operatory, it should be stored in a place not at risk for contamination, such as in a clean drawer or located on a counter *out of the area of spatter contamination.* If you must make notes, use an overglove. If you are using a computer system, the keyboard in the operatory should be barrier-protected between patients. In either case, you can write on a separate scrap piece of paper and later rewrite those notes in the chart outside the operatory. It may also be easier to have another person make entries, provided their hands, or gloves, are not contaminated.

Tips & Hints

- If you do not use an overglove or a sterilizable pen, remember to barrier-protect or clean/disinfect the pen or pencil between patients, and discard any scrap paper in the same manner as contaminated or plain waste, as appropriate.

- If there is anything in the operatory that cannot be removed and is at risk for contamination or aerosolization, and is difficult to clean and disinfect, it must be barrier-protected.

Just as you carefully handle tools and dangerous items at home, the same logic applies to the handling of sharps in the operatory:

- **Never pass sharps in a manner that might injure yourself, another staff member, or the patient.** Announce passes or create a neutral zone.

- **Never recap needles using two hands,** even your own two hands. Use a single-handed "scoop" method or an approved freestanding needle-recapping device or resheathing device.

- **Never disengage a capped needle from a reusable syringe by hand.** Use the disengaging device on the sharps container or appropriate engineering control.

- **Dispose of all nonreusable sharps immediately after use** in a hard-walled, puncture-proof, leak-proof, spill-proof sharps container. Once sharps are placed in the container, they cannot be removed. Sharps containers must be in operatories and at other locations where disposable sharps are generated and used.

Turn handpieces so they face away from you and toward the unit, or cover with a small plastic sheath or protective cover to avoid puncture and scratch injuries from dental burs. Remove all burs immediately after use. Special considerations are necessary to avoid injuring yourself with contaminated instruments:

- **Never wipe debris from instrument tips with gauze held in your hand or with gauze wrapped around your finger.** In addition, you should avoid wiping instruments on your patient's bib. Tape four cotton rolls on the bracket tray cover and wipe debris on these cotton rolls. If you wet one or two of the cotton rolls, it will be easier to clean the instrument tip or blade. You may also use a commercially available product that eliminates the need to hand clean.

- **During procedures with scaling and cutting instruments, never finger rest or fulcrum on the same tooth on which you are working** to avoid pulling a contaminated instrument into your finger.

- **Always grasp instruments by the handle;** never by the working end.

- **Never handle more than one instrument in each hand,** unless trained in assisting techniques for handling two instruments in one hand for instrument transfers.

- **Be especially cautious in handling double-ended instruments.**

4. Segregate Infectious Waste at Chairside

Infectious waste is a major consideration for chairside exposure control. Are paper towels infectious? What about rinse cups? How do you segregate (divide up) and dispose of different types of dental waste?

What is and is not considered infectious waste is defined by federal, state, and local regulations, and will be further discussed in Course #9. According to accepted practices of infection control, *all* medical and dental waste must be handled as if potentially infectious, but may be disposed of in a variety of ways.

Other federal, state, and local authorities regulate the transportation and disposal of infectious waste after it leaves your office. To ensure disposal of the proper items, you should review your Infection Control/Exposure Control Plan for the SOP for "Waste Segregation" in your practice. Once you are familiar with this SOP, and how waste is handled in your practice, you can simply tape a fluid-proof bag or cup to the bracket table and segregate all infectious waste for efficient disposal.

Generally, these items include blood/saliva/serum-soaked gauze, cotton rolls, hard and soft tissue, and contaminated sharps. Infectious waste must be handled and disposed of as a biological hazard (biohazard).

• The disposal of biohazardous waste in your area may be costly, and therefore, the appropriate segregation of waste can save money. Be sure to check with the proper authorities concerning proper disposal procedures. (Chapter #9)

According to your SOP for Segregating Waste list some typical waste items:

Regulated, Biohazard Medical:

_____

_____

_____

Contaminated/Potentially Infectious:

_____

_____

_____

Compliance Evaluation

Evaluating and implementing safe work practices is an ongoing process for everyone in the office. Although there may be regularly scheduled time to introduce safer technology and work habits, staff can work together by observing each other during the day. Any feedback comments should be offered in a way so as to provide valuable suggestions about habits of which you might not be aware. For example, do you ever forget to remove your hand jewelry before gloving and treatment, or leave an operatory with your face mask around your neck? Exposure and infection control should be practiced by everyone, for everyone, and is best managed by team effort and support.

In the morning, the operatory should be cleaned, disinfected, barrier protected (if desired), and prepared for patients. During the day, you must clean, disinfect or change surface barriers, and prepare the operatory in between patients. Following the last patient, remove surface barriers if used and thoroughly clean and disinfect the operatory. This process is known as Operatory Reprocessing.

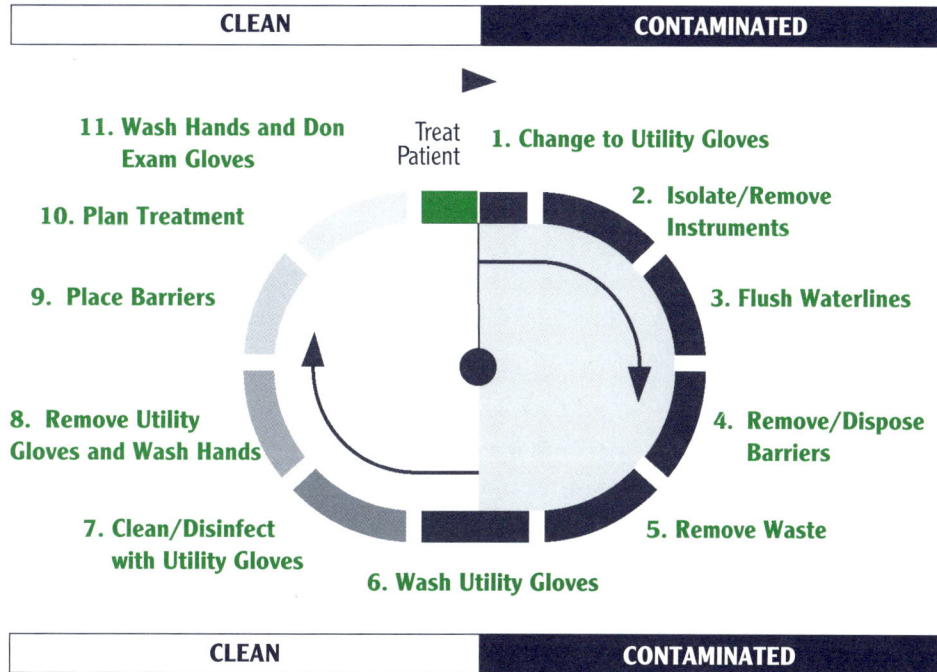

CLEAN	CONTAMINATED

▶

11. Wash Hands and Don Exam Gloves

Treat Patient

1. Change to Utility Gloves

10. Plan Treatment

2. Isolate/Remove Instruments

9. Place Barriers

3. Flush Waterlines

8. Remove Utility Gloves and Wash Hands

4. Remove/Dispose Barriers

7. Clean/Disinfect with Utility Gloves

5. Remove Waste

6. Wash Utility Gloves

CLEAN	CONTAMINATED

Environmental surfaces (i.e., a surface or equipment that does not contact patients directly) can be divided into clinical contact surfaces and housekeeping surfaces. Because housekeeping surfaces (e.g., floors, walls, and sinks) have limited risk of disease transmission, they can be decontaminated with less rigorous methods than those used on dental patient-care items and clinical contact surfaces. Strategies for cleaning and disinfecting surfaces in patient-care areas should consider the potential for direct patient contact, degree and frequency of hand contact, and potential contamination of the surface with body substances, or environmental sources of microorganisms (e.g., soil, dust, or water).

Clinical Contact Surfaces

Clinical contact surfaces can be directly contaminated from patient materials by direct spray or spatter generated during dental procedures, or by contact with the DHCP's gloved hands. These surfaces can subsequently contaminate other instruments, devices, hands, or gloves. Examples of such surfaces include:

- light handles
- dental radiograph equipment
- reusable containers of dental materials
- faucet handles
- pens
- doorknobs
- switches
- dental chairside computers
- drawer handles
- countertops
- telephones

Evidence does not support that housekeeping surfaces (e.g., floors, walls, and sinks) pose a risk for disease transmission in dental healthcare settings. Physical removal of microorganisms and soil by wiping or scrubbing is probably as critical, if not more so, as any antimicrobial effect provided by the agent used. The majority of housekeeping surfaces need to be cleaned only with a detergent and water or an EPA-registered hospital disinfectant/detergent, depending on the nature of the surface and the type and degree of contamination. Always wear the appropriate PPE during decontamination procedures.

Operatory Processing Steps

Cleaning, disinfecting, and barrier-protecting must be accomplished only after instruments are removed for reprocessing, and barriers have been properly removed and disposed. Before beginning, you should be familiar with the SOP for handling and reprocessing contaminated reusable instruments and sharps.

Let's review the process of operatory breakdown and processing, beginning with your first patient of the day:

Prior to first patient

· **Flush air and waterlines for several minutes.**

· **Clean, disinfect or barrier-protect, as appropriate.**

· **Plan treatment needs for the first patient.**

After each patient's treatment

1. **Remove treatment gloves, wash hands, and replace with puncture-resistant utility gloves (see Tips & Hints #2 on following page).**

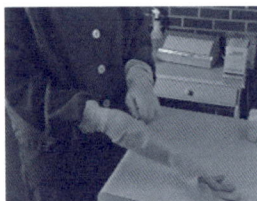

2. **Carefully remove reusable sharps and instruments by placing them in a holding container and transport them in this hard-walled covered container to the instrument reprocessing area.** OSHA states that contaminated reusable sharps shall be placed in containers until processed. The containers shall be puncture-resistant, labeled, and leakproof on the sides and bottom. While there is no requirement for a cover when walking with sharps, the cover protects you and other staff.

3. **Flush air and waterlines for 20-30 seconds, then remove tip, and if disposable, dispose of properly. If reusable, place into the covered transport container.** If this is your last patient, flush the lines for several minutes, then flush the suction lines with cleaner or excess disinfectant, followed by water. If you use "mix-fresh-daily" disinfectant, any left over after the day is the excess disinfectant. Remove and dispose of, or clean and replace, the suction trap basket.

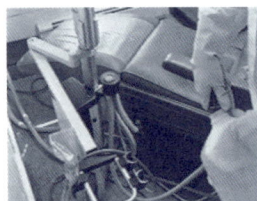

4 & 5 **Remove barriers. Handle as contaminated waste and dispose of this and any other waste appropriately.** (Course #9)

6 **Wash your puncture-resistant utility gloves, because they have been contaminated from the waste and barriers.**

7 **With gloves still on, clean and disinfect surfaces overtly or potentially contaminated that will not be barrier-protected, as specified in the SOP.**

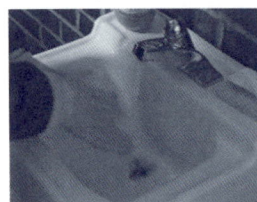

8 **Wash/rinse utility gloves, remove, wash and dry hands, and don new examination gloves.** It is acceptable to use clean, washed hands to replace barriers, as long as you do not touch any items that may be used intraorally.

9 **Replace environmental barriers as outlined in the SOP.** Barriers should not be placed at the end of the day.

10 **Plan treatment needs for the next patient.**

- Clean housekeeping surfaces (e.g., floors, walls, and sinks) with a detergent and water or an EPA-registered hospital disinfectant/detergent on a routine basis, depending on the nature of the surface and type and degree of contamination, and as appropriate, based on the location in the facility, and when visibly soiled.

- Clean mops and cloths after use and allow to dry before reuse; or use single-use, disposable mop heads or cloths.

- Prepare fresh cleaning or EPA-registered disinfecting solutions daily and as instructed by the manufacturer.

- Clean walls, blinds, and window curtains in patient-care areas when they are visibly dusty or soiled.

Tips & Hints

These tips can help make operatory processing proceed quickly and safely:

- Make sure you are wearing the gloves most appropriate for the task. Don't forget to wash utility gloves and remove or replace with clean examination gloves prior to placing barriers.

- Each staff member should have their own puncture-resistant utility gloves that properly fit them and are readily accessible.

- Use other PPE, such as protective eyewear and facemasks, especially with the use of chemicals.

- Disposable barriers should be handled in the same manner as potentially infectious waste, even if they are later disposed of as nonregulated dental waste. This includes nonsharp items such as, covers (barriers), saliva ejectors, and air water syringe tips. If, however, they are overtly contaminated, they will need to be handled and disposed of as infectious waste.

Special Considerations for Radiology

Implementing safe and efficient procedures for exposing and processing X-rays can be especially challenging. To help increase safety for both you and the patient, these procedures deserve special attention.

Most dental practice settings today use digital radiography. It is important to follow the manufacturer's directions for use of the equipment including aseptic management of the digital sensors.

What additional hazards are present while taking and processing X-rays? If your practice uses traditional/non-digital X-rays film, the lead foil, chemical (developer and fixer), and X-ray film each pose potential hazards. Radiation exposure is a less identifiable hazard. Additionally, the potential for contamination exists, as X-rays are usually taken during patient treatment.

Review your procedures for exposing and processing intraoral X-rays and consider the following questions:

- **Where is the exposure button located?**
- **Do you have to leave the operatory to produce the digital image or develop X-ray film?**
- **If you use X-ray film, do you have darkroom equipment and film processors?**
- **How can this be done as efficiently and safely as possible, in order to minimize your risk?**

X-ray Film

As with any regular patient treatment, the appropriate use of PPE is necessary. Always remove gloves and wash hands prior to leaving the exposure or film processing rooms. You'll need to use an overglove, clean gloves or forceps to retrieve items from drawers or the lead-lined X-ray film box to reduce contamination, as well as when pressing the exposure button, if it is not barrier protected for each patient. Because digital sensors or intraoral film have been in the patient's mouth and contaminated with oral fluids, standard precautions must be followed when handling these items.

The process of cleaning, disinfecting and barrier protecting also applies to the exposure of X-rays and the equipment used. Special considerations need to be made for the X-ray tube head, handles, position-indicating device, exposure control settings and exposure button. Carefully review the SOP for exposing and processing X-rays for a list of any specific techniques.

Any waste generated must be disposed as potentially infectious waste. If using X-ray film, the lead foil must be handled according to your state laws. Typically, lead foil needs to be segregated and placed in a labeled lead foil waste container in each processing area to await disposal or recycling by a properly licensed waste hauler.

For further information about infection control methods for digital radiography and other intraoral devices, first review the manufacturer instructions and contact the manufacturer for clarification.

Tips & Hints

- **If you're only taking X-rays, you may use less expensive vinyl gloves in place of latex.**

- **Avoid touching the chair, other surfaces or equipment, to prevent contamination.**

- **When planning X-rays, place film in a sequential order on a tray. Include necessary bitewing tabs, cotton rolls, elastics, and a paper cup for exposed, contaminated X-rays.**

- **Place or tape a waste bag on the countertop in the exposure and processing areas. This can be used for disposal of all waste generated during exposure and processing except for the lead foil from the film packets.**

- **The lead foil should be segregated and placed in a clearly labeled lead foil waste container in each processing area. Course #9 discusses lead foil waste.**

- **Always remove gloves and wash hands prior to removing items from drawers and cabinets, as well as when you leave the exposure and processing rooms. Use clean gloves or overgloves to retrieve items from plastic containers and the lead-lined X-ray film box to avoid contamination. Because the film has been in the patient's mouth, appropriate SOP must be followed.**

Some X-ray film is prepackaged in a protective plastic barrier, which is then removed and discarded after the X-ray exposure is complete. When used appropriately the barrier can be removed from each film in the exposure areas. Careful removal will prevent contamination of the film and reduces the infection control needs for processing.

Special Considerations for the Dental Laboratory

Dental laboratories are integral components of a dental practice, but due to the combination of equipment, chemicals, and potentially infectious waste, labs pose major problems both from occupational exposure risks, and from contamination. Rotary instruments and rag wheels generate particulates and aerosols, which are a hazard to laboratory personnel. Impressions and prostheses that have been inserted into the mouth are contaminated with microorganisms which can be transmitted to personnel via direct contact, or indirectly through aerosols produced during polishing and grinding procedures. Disinfection of these items and the use of personal barriers (masks, gloves, protective eyewear) can effectively reduce this risk. In addition, sterilize rotary instruments and rag wheels between each case, unit dose pumice, barrier-protect the pumice pan, and use the safety shield provided for the lathe.

Disinfection of Laboratory Items

The CDC and ADA have recommended that all saliva-contaminated items be rinsed with water and disinfected prior to sending to a laboratory. This includes impressions, prostheses, wax bites, etc. In addition, items returned from a laboratory must be disinfected prior to delivery to the patient.

Impressions and prostheses should be rinsed under running water to remove visible debris, then disinfected in a manner that won't damage the material, yet provides adequate disinfection. You should consult the manufacturer's directions for the recommended disinfectant and optimal disinfection/sterilization procedures. Be aware that residual chemicals often remain on prostheses and impressions after they've been disinfected or sterilized, so it is important to thoroughly rinse all materials before they are replaced in a patient's mouth.

Tips & Hints

- **Your practice should communicate with any dental laboratories used regarding precautions taken for infection control. This prevents duplication of effort and reduces the risk of distortion or damage from exposure to disinfectant solutions. A written agreement should be developed with any outside laboratory the practice may use. The agreement should cover infection control policy, and procedures for material sent to and returned from the lab.**

The same guidelines for the use of PPE, cleaning, disinfecting, and barrier-protection also apply to in-house laboratories. Since laboratories are full of equipment and chemicals, everything should be labeled with the appropriate safety warnings and signs. Care must be taken with in-office adjustments to prevent contamination of prostheses when making adjustments. The use of sterilized or disposable rag wheels and unit doses of polishing compounds will prevent contamination of prostheses and the need for multiple disinfections with repeat try-ins. Finally, you should keep the following in mind:

- **Don't eat, drink, smoke, or apply cosmetics in the lab.**
- **Lab refrigerators should store medical and dental materials only and should not be used for storage of food or beverages.**

Sterile/Disposable rag wheels   **Unit dosed amounts**

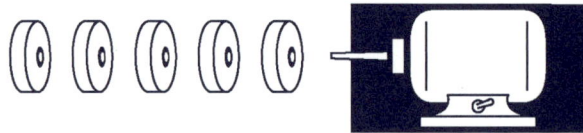

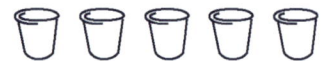

- **Use unit-dosed polishing compounds, sterilized or disposable rag wheels, and disposable tray liners to prevent contamination of prostheses and multiple-disinfection cycles for repeat try-ins.**

Standard Operating Procedures

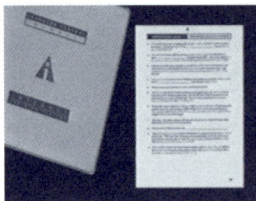

Maintaining an aseptic environment poses a challenge to your daily work life. But, using a combination of logic, time management, and various exposure control principles, it is possible to reach this goal safely and efficiently. To further expand your understanding of the practice's policies and techniques, review the following SOPs which are practice-specific:

- **Operatory processing**
- **The exposure of radiographs - film and digital sensors**
- **Film processing**
- **Dental Office Laboratory**
- **Other SOPs your practice may have specific to daily procedures**

Discussion

Discuss with your Infection Control Coordinator or Safety Officer the specific standard operating procedures for daily infection control procedures.

Objectives

Upon completion of this course on instrument reprocessing, you will be able to:

1. Identify 10 steps in instrument reprocessing.

2. Differentiate three infection-control categories (Spaulding classification) of patient care items.

3. Explain engineering controls and work practices used to prevent exposure when handling, transporting and packaging contaminated instruments.

4. Describe two methods of cleaning instruments.

5. Explain the function of packaging in instrument reprocessing and storage.

6. Identify six methods of sterilization.

7. Explain three ways to increase sterilization efficiency.

8. Compare and contrast three methods of monitoring sterilization.

9. Explain why dental handpieces should be heat-sterilized between patient/client uses.

10. Demonstrate effective instrument reprocessing.

Focus

During Course #4 you focused on operatory preparation and processing to provide as aseptic an environment as possible. In this course, you will address this goal from the perspective of cleaning and sterilizing reusable instruments, a process referred to as "instrument reprocessing" or "instrument recirculation."

How Instrument Reprocessing Effects Operatory Processing

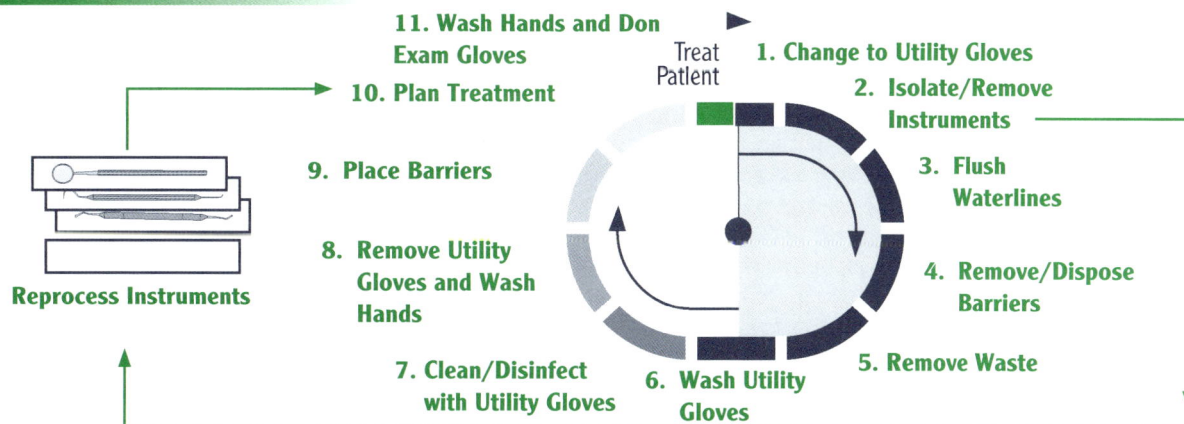

Treat Patient

11. Wash Hands and Don Exam Gloves

10. Plan Treatment

9. Place Barriers

8. Remove Utility Gloves and Wash Hands

7. Clean/Disinfect with Utility Gloves

Reprocess Instruments

1. Change to Utility Gloves

2. Isolate/Remove Instruments

3. Flush Waterlines

4. Remove/Dispose Barriers

5. Remove Waste

6. Wash Utility Gloves

Instrument reprocessing is a major component of any exposure control program. While preparing instruments for sterilization, there is a potential for an exposure incident or injury. And if you are using improperly sterilized instruments, you and your patients are at risk for contamination. It is important to establish an aseptic environment for the health and safety of you and your patients. Like operatory processing, instrument reprocessing requires an assessment of needs to establish methods of management and efficiency. Instrument reprocessing involves the following steps:

- **Handling contaminated instruments**
- **Isolating contaminated instruments for transport in a transport container**
- **Temporarily placing instruments in a container with a holding solution, when immediate cleaning is not possible**
- **Instrument cleaning**
- **Packaging and labeling**
- **Sterilization and monitoring procedures**
- **Storage of packaged sterile items**
- **Batch tracking or quality control for sterilization**
  - Processing of unused, expired packages
  - Tracking the load by number and date for inventory control and in case of a biologic monitoring failure

Instrument Reprocessing

For these reasons, instrument reprocessing must be well-planned and organized. Your practice's Infection Control/Exposure Control Plan should contain SOPs for reprocessing instruments with set procedures, designated tasks, and monitoring records.

Procedures for reprocessing depend on the type of instrument and how it is used. In dentistry, there are three classifications of items that are used during patient treatment. This is also known as the Spaulding Classification System.

Infection-Control Categories of Patient-Care Items (Spaulding Classification)

Category	Definition	Dental Instrument or Item
Critical	**Penetrates soft tissue, contacts bone, enters into or contacts the bloodstream or other normally sterile tissue**	**Surgical instruments, periodontal scalers, scalpel blades, surgical dental burs**
Semicritical	**Contacts mucous membranes or non-intact skin; will not penetrate soft tissue, contact bone, enter into or contact the blood stream or other normally sterile tissue**	**Dental mouth mirror, amalgam condenser, reusable dental impression trays, dental handpieces***
Noncritical	**Contacts intact skin**	**Radiograph head/cone, blood pressure cuff, facebow, pulse oximeter**

* Although dental handpieces are considered a semicritical item, they should always be heat-sterilized between uses and not high-level disinfected.

**1.
Treatment**

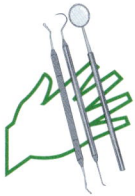

The assessment needs for reprocessing are similar to the assessment needs described in Course #4. First, identify potential hazards to you and your patients. Next, select engineering controls and/or develop work practice controls to help reduce or avoid these hazards. Some questions you may consider:

- **During clinical procedures, where do you place contaminated instruments?**
- **What do you do with instruments when you are finished with treatment?**
- **How do you dispose of single-use contaminated sharps?**
- **Do you use any additional protective equipment when handling these items?**

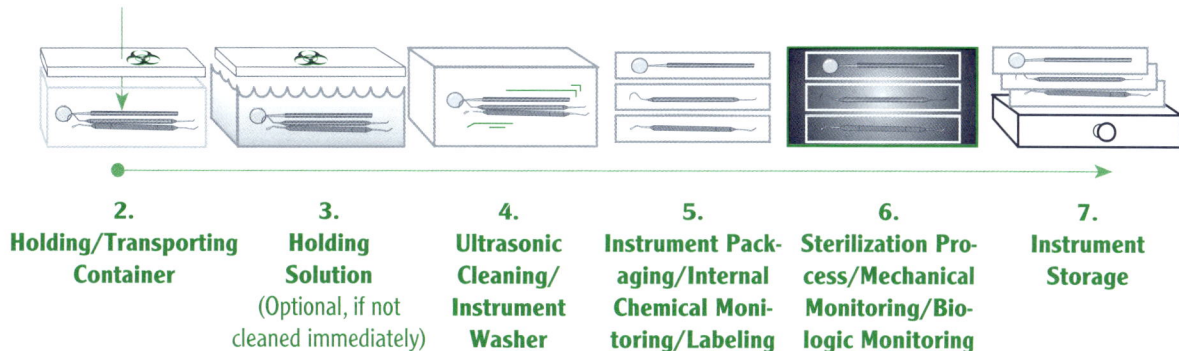

| **2.**
Holding/Transporting
Container | **3.**
Holding
Solution
(Optional, if not
cleaned immediately) | **4.**
Ultrasonic
Cleaning/
Instrument
Washer | **5.**
Instrument Pack-
aging/Internal
Chemical Moni-
toring/Labeling | **6.**
Sterilization Pro-
cess/Mechanical
Monitoring/Bio-
logic Monitoring | **7.**
Instrument
Storage |

Following treatment, reusable instruments go through a sterilization process, while single-use sharps must be properly isolated and discarded. The cycle, as outlined above, provides a safe, time-efficient method for reprocessing instruments.

CDC recommends that your practice have manufacturer instructions for reprocessing reusable dental instruments and equipment readily available in or near your instrument reprocessing area. Open your practice's Infection Control/Exposure Control Plan to the SOP for Instrument Reprocessing and use it as a reference during this course.

Handling Contaminated Instruments

A basic element for controlling chairside exposure during patient treatment procedures is to reduce the risk of exposure incidents from contaminated sharps. This caution must be applied to instrument reprocessing after treatment, where there is a potential for injury. *During* treatment, follow the recommendations for reducing the potential for an exposure incident when handling sharps, as presented in Course #4. *Following* treatment, reusable critical and semicritical instruments go through a sterilization process, while single-use or disposable instruments and items must be properly handled, isolated, and discarded as contaminated in a sharps container (Course #9).

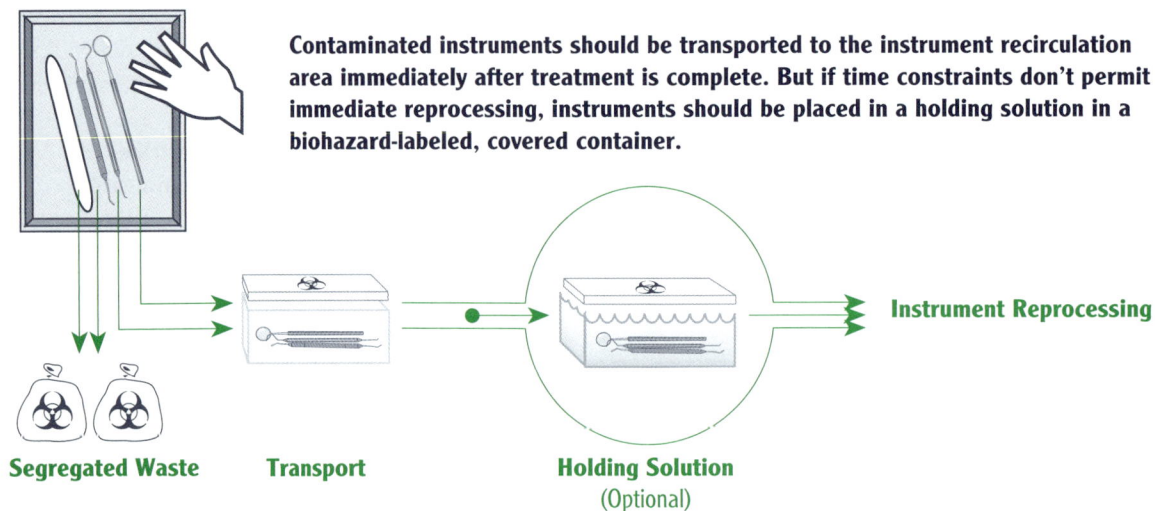

Contaminated instruments should be transported to the instrument recirculation area immediately after treatment is complete. But if time constraints don't permit immediate reprocessing, instruments should be placed in a holding solution in a biohazard-labeled, covered container.

Segregated Waste   **Transport**   **Holding Solution**
(Optional)

Instrument Reprocessing

Transporting Instruments

Transporting or moving instruments can be done with something as simple as a solid plastic container with a lid. Instruments are placed in the container in the operatory, covered, and carried to the reprocessing area. OSHA requires a transport container that is puncture-resistant, leakproof with solid sides and bottom, and displays a biohazard label. OSHA does not require a lid; however, CDC recommends a covered container to minimize exposure potential while walking with sharps.

While transporting contaminated instruments, remember to:

- **Wear appropriate PPE.** Wear puncture-resistant, heavy-duty utility gloves (in place of treatment/examination gloves) to reduce the risk of injury.

- **Isolate and cover instruments.** Instruments should be placed in an appropriate transport-container at the point of use to prevent percutaneous injuries during transport to the instrument reprocessing area. When transporting instruments to the reprocessing area, a covered container with solid sides and bottom minimizes the primary risk of puncture injury to your self, your patients, and staff. A biohazard label should be on the outside of the container.

- Never transport contaminated instruments in a solution.

Tips & Hints

- **If your setting uses ultrasonic cleaning, consider purchasing several baskets for your ultrasonic cleaner. Use one of these, together with a larger transport container, to safely transport instruments from the operatory to a holding container and/ or to the ultrasonic cleaner. This will facilitate safe and efficient transport between containers.**

In your practice, what is used to contain instruments during cleanup and transport?

_____

_____

_____

Are instruments in your practice immediately cleaned and packaged after use, or are they placed in a holding solution or storage area to be reprocessed later?

_____

Who is responsible for each step of reprocessing?

_____

Where are the puncture-resistant gloves kept?

_____

Holding Solutions

Have you ever left dirty dishes to sit at home without rinsing or soaking them? If you have, you know that it is much harder to clean them later. The same is true of dental instruments. If instruments cannot be cleaned immediately after patient treatment, they can be placed in a holding solution. As with your dishes at home, by keeping instruments moist, debris can't dry and harden. This makes the cleaning process much more effective. Later, when you have time, you can begin the actual reprocessing of the instruments. The holding solution should be a simple detergent and water, not an immersion disinfectant/sterilant.

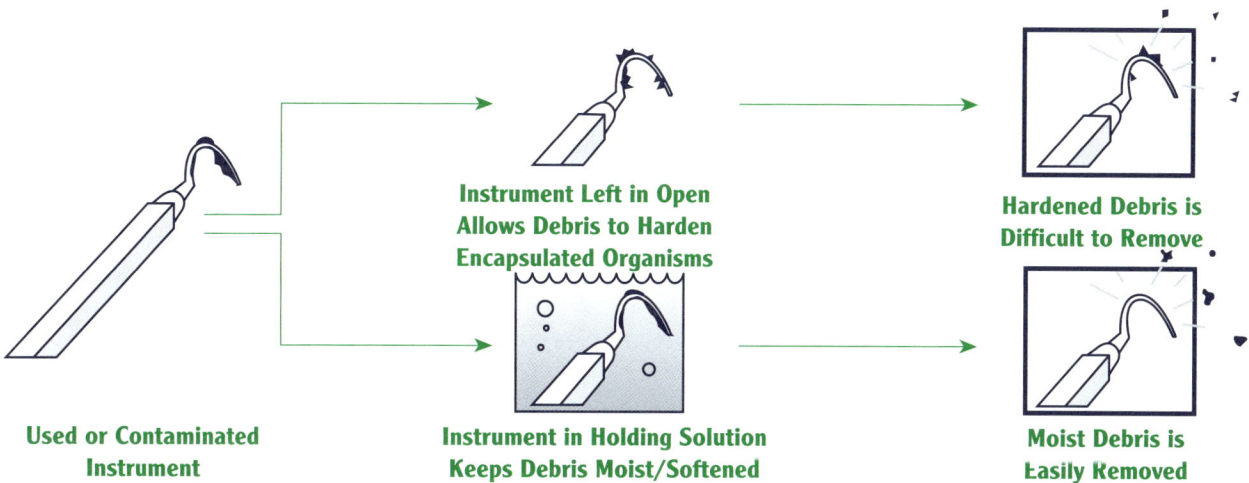

Used or Contaminated Instrument

Instrument Left in Open Allows Debris to Harden Encapsulated Organisms

Hardened Debris is Difficult to Remove

Instrument in Holding Solution Keeps Debris Moist/Softened

Moist Debris is Easily Removed

A holding container with solution should be placed in the reprocessing area. Instruments should be transported from the operatory to this area in a transport container with solid bottom and side walls. Once in the reprocessing area, the holding solution can be used if the instruments are to be reprocessed later.

Note:

· **You can use the holding container, without solution, to transport instruments to the reprocessing area and then add the presoak holding solution. Do not transport instruments using a holding container with solution. To prevent spilling of solution which may be contaminated, do not walk with liquids.**

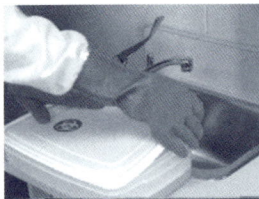

A holding solution is simply a noncorrosive liquid, preferably one that contains a surfactant, stored in a hard-walled, spill-proof container with a lid. Because of the potential exposure to infectious material, the container must be labeled as a biohazard. It is not cost-effective nor necessary to use a disinfectant as the holding solution, because contaminated particles on the instruments prevent effective disinfection. In addition, the chemical becomes contaminated with bioburden, rendering the disinfectant ineffective over time. Remember that a holding solution is used only as a way to keep debris moist to facilitate cleaning later. If instruments are cleaned soon after transport to the reprocessing area, there is no need to place them in a holding solution/container.

Change Solution Twice a Day

How often should you change a holding solution? Twice a day is acceptable, or more often if it looks visibly contaminated or cloudy. At the same time, you should also take the opportunity to clean and disinfect the holding container itself. Always wear appropriate PPE when handling the container due to the contamination of the container and solution.

Notes:

- The holding solution must be treated as contaminated. When cleaning out the holding container and after emptying holding solution into a sink, you must also clean and disinfect the sink.
- Instruments should be reprocessed as soon as possible after use and not left in holding solutions for extended periods of time.
- Holding solutions are not necessary if instruments are cleaned soon after use.

Tips & Hints

- Use a commercial medical non-corrosive cleaning solution or dishwasher detergent for your holding solution. Detergents designed for household dishwashers are low-foaming and are available as low cost powders and liquids at any supermarket. Dishwasher detergents contain surfactant and anti-corrosive agents. Because a dishwasher detergent will be used in a healthcare employment setting and more often than in a typical household, you must contact the manufacturer for a Safety Data Sheet (SDS) which must be on file. (Course #8)

Instrument Cleaning

Two methods of instrument cleaning are considered acceptable: automated and manual. Automated methods include the use of ultrasonic cleaners and instrument washers. Hand scrubbing is a manual way of cleaning instruments. Automated methods are preferred over hand scrubbing because they reduce your contact with contaminated instruments and in turn, the chance of exposure.

Preliminary Steps

With each method, you must wear your PPE until items are packaged. Loose instruments should only be removed from the holding container using forceps or a transfer basket. After removal from holding solution, rinse the items under running water to remove residual holding solution and any loose debris.

Hand Scrubbing

If your office does not use automated cleaning equipment (e.g., ultrasonic, thermal disinfector or medical instrument washer) instruments may be cleaned by hand. Because of the risks involved with hand scrubbing, special precautions must be observed to reduce the chance of an exposure incident.

Note:

Check with your state regulations to see if there are any restrictions on hand scrubbing instruments. You may be required to use safer cleaning processes and devices.

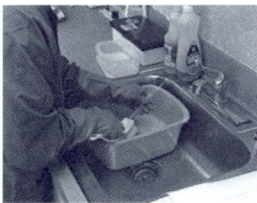

Details on hand scrubbing, if used, are outlined in your practice's SOP, but these suggestions will help make hand scrubbing safer:

- **Wear appropriate barriers, including eyewear, mask, and puncture-resistant gloves.** Do not remove the PPE until all of the items have been cleaned and are appropriately packaged.

- **Clean only two to three instruments at a time.**

- **Scrub instruments low in the sink under running water, using a long-handled or wide-surface brush and a detergent that is noncorrosive.** Use the brush in a manner that helps protect your hand from the sharp instruments while scrubbing.

- **Inspect all instruments for remaining debris**; if necessary, scrub again.

- **Dry instruments by allowing them to air dry or by carefully patting with several thicknesses of toweling; don't rub.** Instruments can then be divided into procedure-oriented groups and packaged for sterilization.

Ultrasonic Cleaning

Using a detergent solution and sonic-action, ultrasonic cleaners break up and loosen debris on instruments. To maintain efficiency, ultrasonic cleaners must undergo scheduled maintenance and function tests, according to the manufacturer's directions. Ultimately, however, it is your responsibility to maintain the efficiency of the ultrasonic cleaners.

- **Always follow the manufacturer's directions for use, solutions, and maintenance.** The manufacturer will also indicate how much solution to put into the tank, as well as cycle times for loose instruments versus cassettes.

- **Test cleaning solution for effectiveness.** For most units, immerse a strip of aluminum foil that is at least 2" wide and 3" long in the cleaner for exactly 20 seconds. Then, hold the foil to light to check for an even distribution of dents or small holes. If none exist, the cleaner isn't working. This is called a "function" test. You should check with the manufacturer of your ultrasonic cleaner for precise directions since function test directions and methods may differ from one manufacturer to another.

- **Don't overload the tank.** Place the instruments or cassettes in a cleaning basket. This prevents having to reach into the contaminated solution later to retrieve the cleaned items. The number of items the basket can safely hold will vary with size of the basket, and whether instruments are loose or in a cassette.

- **Only use solutions formulated for use in the ultrasonic bath.** Other chemicals, such as disinfectants, may create the potential for hazardous fumes.

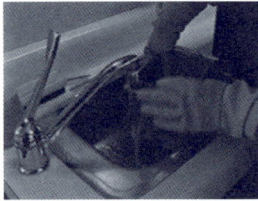

- **Rinse instruments or cassettes both before and after the cycle.** This is especially true for instruments that were in a holding solution. You do not want to transfer holding solution to the ultrasonic cleaner.

- **Once the cycle is complete, allow the instruments to air dry or pat them dry with several thicknesses of toweling.** Instruments can then be divided into procedure-oriented groups and packaged for sterilization.

- **When using ultrasonic cleaners there are other factors to take into account, such as preventing contamination if the ultrasonic cleaner is used to clean both instruments and prostheses.** Consult your SOP for further information about these special considerations.

- **Follow the manufacturer's directions for your specific equipment and solutions and always keep the cover on the tank while running.**

Thermal Disinfection/Instrument Washers

A medical instrument washer or thermal disinfector looks like a dishwasher and works on a similar principle. However, they are FDA-cleared medical devices designed to clean medical/dental instruments. A thermal disinfector achieves a high-level of disinfection. It is, however, not a sterilizer and all critical and semi-critical items still need to be packaged and sterilized. An additional benefit of some of the instrument washers is that instruments are dry when the cycle is completed, immediately ready to be packaged for sterilization.

Use only thermal washer/disinfectors that are designed for use in healthcare settings. In the US, these must be cleared by the FDA. Follow the manufacturer's maintenance and function test directions.

Packaging of Reusable Instruments

Clean instruments are not the same as *sterile* instruments. Clean simply means free of gross debris. Instruments must be packaged and sterilized before being used on a patient. Packaging serves two purposes:

1. **Proper storage:** The packaging provides a barrier for instruments after sterilization (unpackaged sterilized instruments are at a greater risk for contamination prior to patient use than packaged instruments).

2. **Record Keeping:** All packaged instruments should be labeled with the date of sterilization, the cycle number, and the type of instruments they contain (unless the packaging is see-through), the name or initials of the "packager," and any other practice-specific information (see your SOP for packaging). If multiple sterilizers are used in the facility, add the name or number of the sterilizer used on the outside of the packaging material to facilitate the retrieval of reprocessed items in the event of a sterilization failure.

Tips & Hints

- Packaging paper becomes less flexible after a sterilization cycle. The force of a pen or pencil after sterilization could possibly pierce the packaging. All labeling should be done before sterilization.

- Hinged instruments should be packaged in the open or unnotched position.

Sterilization of unwrapped instruments is generally not recommended due to the risk of contaminating the items after sterilization. The following is recommended if you must sterilize unwrapped instruments: This technique, formerly known as *flash sterilization*, is now termed *immediate-use sterilization*. This term means that an item is steam sterilized for a specific patient and procedure, used immediately when removed from the sterilizer, and not stored for future use. Immediate-use sterilization may be used when there is an urgent need, such as when an important instrument is dropped during treatment and no replacement is available. Immediate-use sterilization should not be used to save time or money spent on wrapping, or as an alternative to purchasing multiple sets of instruments. When using this method of sterilization:

1. **Clean and dry instruments before the unwrapped sterilization cycle.**
2. **Use mechanical and chemical indicators for each unwrapped sterilization cycle** (i.e., place a chemical indicator among the instruments or items to be sterilized).
3. **Allow unwrapped instruments to dry and cool in the sterilizer before they are handled to avoid contamination and thermal injury.**
4. **Semicritical instruments that will be used immediately or within a short time can be sterilized unwrapped on a tray or in a container system, provided that the instruments are handled aseptically during removal from the sterilizer and immediately transported to the point of use.**
5. **Critical instruments intended for immediate reuse can be sterilized unwrapped if the instruments are maintained sterile during removal from the sterilizer and transported to the point of use** (e.g., transported in a sterile covered container).
6. **Do not use immediate-use sterilization for implantable devices.**
7. **Keep sterilized instruments packaged/wrapped until the point of use.**

In dentistry, implantable devices are sterilized by the manufacturer and do not need to be re-sterilized before use if handled according to the device manufacturer's instructions. If the sterility of an implantable device is compromised, the device should not be used and should be replaced by a new manufacturer-sterilized implantable device.

Packaging materials and techniques depend on the type of sterilization equipment used. Check your practice's SOP and the directions provided by the manufacturer of the sterilization equipment you use for the correct packaging materials.

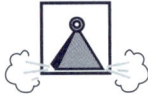

STERILIZER	PACKAGING MATERIALS
Steam Heat under Pressure (Autoclave)	Paper, paper-plastic peel pouches, heat-resistant plastic, surgical muslin, wrapped perforated metal cassettes. Solid closed metal containers and sealed glass containers are not acceptable.
Dry Heat/Dry Heat Oven Rapid Heat Transfer	Paper bags (approved for dry heat), muslin, aluminum foil, wrapped cassettes, trays or metal pans. Due to high temperatures, plastics are not acceptable.
Unsaturated Chemical Vapor (Chemiclave)	Wrapped perforated metal cassettes, paper, paper-plastic peel pouches. Solid closed metal containers and sealed glass jars are not acceptable.
Ethylene Oxide	Paper or plastic bags. Since the gas needs to permeate to the instruments, sealed metal or glass is not acceptable.

Packaging Considerations

When packaging instruments, there are many factors that are specific to your practice and the type of sterilizer and packaging material used. Using your SOP for packaging, answer the following question:

According to your SOP, what information should you write on each package/label before sterilization?

_____

_____

Cassettes

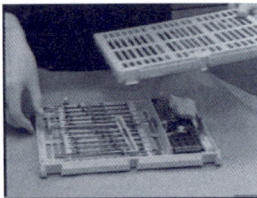

A system that simplifies the entire reprocessing cycle, including packaging, is the use of cassettes during the treatment, holding, cleaning, sterilization, and storage of instruments. A cassette is a lockable container designed to hold all or part of the instruments required for a specific clinical procedure, and is made out of either metal or hard resin/plastic. Instruments remain in the cassette during treatment, with clinicians working out of the cassette. After a procedure is completed, the clinician checks to see that the instruments are properly seated in the cassette, which is then closed and locked in the operatory, transported to the reprocessing area, and placed directly into an ultrasonic cleaner or instrument washer. The cassette is not a transport container, because it has holes on the bottom and sides. The cassette should be placed in a solid bottom, side-walled container displaying a biohazard label for transport from the operatory to the instrument processing area.

Even if you use cassettes, it is recommended to still use a transport container with solid sides and bottom.

After appropriate cleaning and drying, the cassette is opened and loaded with new, single-use items such as gauze and cotton rolls for the specified procedure. The cassette is then closed, covered with barrier wrap, labeled, and sterilized. After sterilization, the packaged cassette is stored until needed. The cassette barrier wrap may also be used as a tray cover during treatment. The advantages of cassettes include:

- **reduced hand contact with contaminated instruments,**
- **reduced wear and tear on the instruments themselves, and**
- **procedure organization.**

Cassettes can improve both efficiency and safety.

There are also cassettes, or instrument baskets, that are simply small containers with a lid and holes. These cassettes simplify the first part of the reprocessing cycle. Contaminated instruments are placed into the cassette in the operatory. The cassette is closed and placed into the transport container. After transporting to the reprocessing area, the cassette is placed into the ultrasonic cleaner. It is only after cleaning, and air-drying that the cassette is opened and instruments inspected and packaged for sterilizing.

Dental Sterilization Methods

Sterilization goes beyond disinfection to destroy *all* microbial forms, including bacterial endospores. **NOTE:** Even though the goal of sterilization is to kill all living microorganisms, there is a specific manufacturing standard for sterilization called the Sterility Assurance Level (SAL). In practical terms, this is expressed as the probability of a surviving microorganism on an item as being 1 in 1 million (source: Comprehensive Guide to steam Sterilization and Sterility assurance in healthcare facilities. ANSI/AAMI ST79 2010 & A1: 2010, A2:2011, A3: 2012, 2017). The concept of sterilization is simple and there are various methods of accomplishing sterilization. Heat sterilization is considered the most effective method in dentistry, particularly when combined with steam or unsaturated chemical vapor under pressure. Your practice may use one or a combination of sterilization methods, so you should consult the Infection Control/Exposure Control Plan for the SOP on how to use the sterilizing equipment in your practice.

Six methods of Sterilization:

It is helpful to understand the different types of sterilization methods and equipment available, regardless of which method is used in your practice.

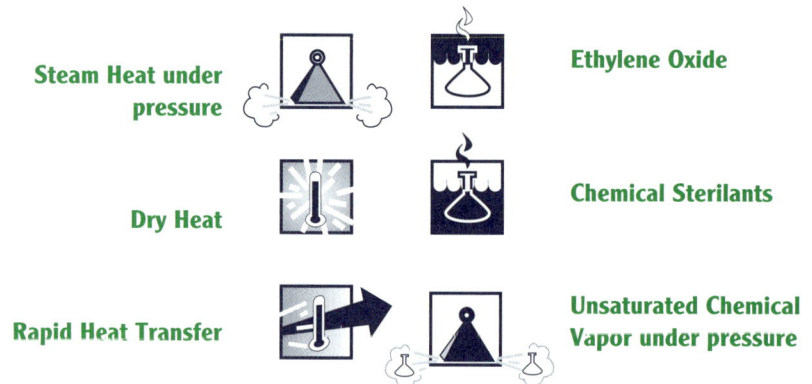

Steam Heat under pressure

Ethylene Oxide

Dry Heat

Chemical Sterilants

Rapid Heat Transfer

Unsaturated Chemical Vapor under pressure

Note:

Packaged instruments must be placed in the sterilizer so the sterilizing medium can access all of the packages. If the sterilizer is overloaded, there may be packages with cold spots, which can result in incomplete sterilization. If your practice's sterilizer has a basket type of loading device instead of several trays, packages should be layered in alternating vertical and horizontal rows to prevent cold spots and to allow the sterilizing medium to penetrate all of the packages.

1. Steam Heat Under Pressure

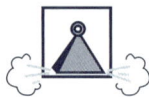

Sterilization of critical and semi-critical instruments is most effectively accomplished by heat methods. High temperature methods include steam (e.g. autoclave), dry heat, or chemical vapor. These methods are intended for use on critical and semi-critical items that are heat tolerant.

Sterilization using saturated steam heat under pressure is the most frequently used method in the U.S. The heat and steam pressure are quite effective in killing microorganisms, including bacterial endospores. Sterilizers that use steam heat under pressure are commonly known as *autoclaves*.

Advantages of the autoclave include:
- **Its compatibility with a wide variety of packaging materials and dental devices, including heat-resistant plastics, dental handpieces, and cotton and cloth material items, such as gauze and cotton rolls.**
- **It uses distilled water to produce steam, which poses fewer hazards than the chemicals used in unsaturated chemical vapor sterilizers.**

A drawback of sterilization using steam heat under pressure is that the moisture may cause corrosion on certain high-carbon steel products.

It's important to remove air from an autoclave chamber during the sterilization process so that the chamber will be saturated with steam. Any air pockets remaining in the chamber will not reach sterilization temperatures.

There are two types of steam autoclaves based on how the chamber air is removed:
- **Gravity displacement**
- **Dynamic air-removal**

Gravity displacement steam autoclaves, once the most common type of tabletop autoclave used in dentistry, relies on gravity for downward air displacement to remove air from the sterilization chamber. Generally, wrapped instruments are sterilized at temperatures reaching 250°F (121°C).

For dynamic air-removal steam sterilizers, a mechanical vacuum pump removes air from the sterilizer chamber to enhance drying. This results in shorter cycles compared with gravity displacement autoclaves. Generally, wrapped instruments are sterilized with dynamic air-removal systems at 270°F (132°C). Dynamic air-removal steam sterilizers include pre-vacuum steam autoclaves and steam-flush pressure-pulse autoclaves.

Sterility may be compromised if instrument packages are removed from an autoclave before the drying cycle is complete. Always refer to the manufacturer's instructions for proper use and care of your sterilizer.

Note:

"Flash" sterilization is an outdated term for a method of sterilization where instruments are placed unwrapped into a steam sterilizer. Today, the term is "Immediate-Use Steam Sterilization" and means that the item is used promptly upon removal from the sterilizer, for a specific patient and procedure, and not stored for future use. Unwrapped sterile instruments can pose an infection control challenge. For additional information, see "Recommendations for Unwrapped Instruments" discussed previously in this course and the CDC Guidelines for Infection Control in Dental Health-Care Settings, 2003.

Tips & Hints

· **Tap water, or nondistilled water, may contain impurities that can corrode carbon steel products and harm internal components of your autoclave. To help prevent corrosion be sure that you use distilled water and thoroughly dry instruments before packaging, to remove any tap water if rinsing is required prior to sterilization.**

· **Mixing carbon steel products with stainless steel products may pit the stainless steel. It is recommended that you separate these metals in different packs or, better yet, use different autoclave cycles.**

· **Items that have a tendency to corrode or dull in an autoclave can also be treated with an anticorrosive dip or spray prior to packaging for steam autoclaving.**

2. Dry Heat (Static-Air)

Dry heat sterilizers work on the principle of using high temperatures (320°F or 160°C) to kill all microorganisms. Since steam is not used, dry heat sterilizers require even higher temperatures than autoclaves to be effective. This method, therefore, is not suitable for materials, such as some plastics and handpieces that cannot withstand high temperatures. Dry heat does not corrode or dull cutting instruments, as may occur with an autoclave. The process is slower than steam heat sterilizing, as it takes between one and two hours, depending on the temperature used.

3. Rapid Heat Transfer (Forced Air)

Another method of dry heat sterilization, known as "rapid heat transfer," utilizes a much higher temperature (375°F or 190°C) and forced air to sterilize instruments more quickly. With this method, loose items may be sterilized in about six minutes and packaged items in about 12 minutes. Loose items pose an aseptic challenge, as they cannot be aseptically stored and must either be used or packaged immediately after sterilization. This method is best for sterilizing instruments while a patient is in the operatory. As with dry heat, special attention needs to be paid to the types of instruments being sterilized, as some plastic materials cannot withstand the higher temperatures of rapid heat transfer.

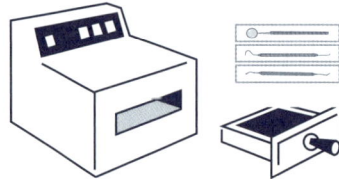

Rapid Heat Transfer uses circulating high temperature air to sterilize instruments quickly.

4. Unsaturated Chemical Vapor

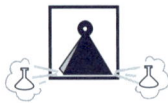

Unsaturated chemical vapor sterilizers combine heat, pressure, and various chemicals to produce a layer of condensed chemicals on the instruments, which in turn kills microorganisms. The temperature and pressure are greater than that used in an autoclave. Items must be completely dry prior to sterilization to prevent corrosion from the exposure to the chemicals.

Because chemicals are used (0.23% formaldehyde, 72.38% ethanol, in addition to acetone, ketone, water and other alcohols), there is some concern about fumes being released during sterilization, especially when the heat chamber door is opened at the end of the cycle. Proper room ventilation, combined with a built-in purging system, reduces the release of vapor into the work area. Never open the door of the sterilizer before completion of the purge cycle. Consult the manufacturer's directions for use and applicable hazard communication and management requirements.

5. Ethylene Oxide

Ethylene oxide is a chemical gas, which, as in unsaturated chemical vapor sterilizers, coats instruments with a film that sterilizes the instruments.

Ethylene oxide does have its disadvantages, making it less practical to use in a dental practice. These disadvantages include:

- **Ethylene oxide is potentially explosive, so packaged instruments are placed in a special container, called a "spark shield," in a well-ventilated area for the sterilization cycle. The venting requirements are particularly extensive.**

- **The cycle time, including venting, may vary from 10 to 48 hours,** depending on the material.

- **All items must be sufficiently ventilated to remove all residual vapors, as the gas can cause painful burns on human tissues.**

Chemical sterilants are considered medical devices and must be cleared for market by the FDA. These are capable of killing spore-forming organisms when used in the appropriate manner and in accordance with the product's label claims. There are, however, significant limitations:

- **Items cannot be packaged for reprocessing.**
- **Biologic monitoring of the process is not possible; sterilization cannot be verified.**
- **Certain items may not be compatible with chemical sterilants.**
- **The chemical must be mixed, stored and used according to the manufacturer's instructions. Close monitoring of the chemical is necessary to ensure appropriate concentration and stability.** This requires test-strips and additional time to maintain records.
- **Items must remain immersed in the chemical undisturbed for the designated time.** This may, for example, require 10 hours of undisturbed immersion.
- **These chemicals may pose health risks and are known sensitizers.**
- **Cleaning is critical. The chemical is affected by bioburden and may become ineffective.**
- **After removing items from chemicals, thoroughly rinse with sterile water.**

Chemical sterilants may be the preferred method of sterilization for semicritical items that cannot withstand exposure to heat or ethylene oxide, but in general, they are not practical for most items, nor are they appropriate for critical items.

Note:

Glass Bead and Salt Sterilizers are not FDA-cleared sterilizers. Bead sterilizers have been used in dentistry to reprocess small metallic instruments (e.g., endodontic files). FDA has determined that a risk of infection exists with these devices because of their potential failure to sterilize dental instruments and has required their commercial distribution cease unless the manufacturer files a premarket approval application. If a bead sterilizer is employed, DHCP assume the risk of employing a dental device FDA has deemed neither safe nor effective.

After Sterilization

Once sterilization and drying cycles are complete, slowly open the sterilizer door. Next, carefully remove the packages from the sterilizer. To avoid burns and injuries, you should wear heat-resistant gloves, such as oven mitts, and depending on your sterilizer, protective eyewear and a face mask (for protection against steam or chemical vapor).

Storage of Sterile Instruments

All sterile instruments should remain packaged for storage. Proper storage areas include cabinets or drawers that are clean, dry, and closeable. The shelf life of packaged sterile dental instruments is dependent upon the integrity of the packaging material and the storage environment. If the storage area is constantly opened, you may want to reduce the safe storage time. Storage areas should be cleaned on a routine basis and checked daily to see if the area is clean and dry. Other recommendations include:

- **Store sterile items and dental supplies in covered or closed cabinets, if possible**
- **Use date or event-related shelf-life for storage of wrapped, sterilized instruments and devices**
- **Examine wrapped packages of sterilized instruments before opening them to ensure the barrier wrap has not been compromised during storage**
- **Reclean, repack, and resterilize any instrument package that has been compromised**
- **Open packaged instruments in front of patients to visually demonstrate that the instruments have been reprocessed**

Sterilization Equipment Parameters

Use the manufacturer's instructions/directions for use to fill out the table below. (The first space is filled out with an example.)

- **Enter the brand name and model number of each sterilizer, as well as the sterilization method described earlier.**

- **If you treat some instruments differently by using different temperatures, pressures or times, use a separate row for each treatment.**

Sterilizer Name and Method	LOAD items to be sterilized	Exposure Time	Temperature °F	Pressure PSI	Dry/Cool Time
Steam Autoclave (EXAMPLE)	Packaged Instruments	30 min.	250° F (121°C)	16-18	30 min.
Sterilizer #1					
Sterilizer #2					
Sterilizer #3					

Increasing Sterilization Efficiency

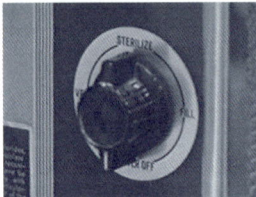

The ultimate goal of instrument reprocessing is to sterilize all of your instruments all of the time, and to have them remain sterile until they are needed for use during patient treatment. Although there is no way to absolutely guarantee sterilization (unless each package is biologic monitored), the following suggestions will help increase the effectiveness and ease of the process:

- **Follow manufacturer's instructions including validated reprocessing directions.**

- **Leave hinged instruments open to allow the sterilizing agent to contact all areas of the instrument.**

- **Don't overload the packages or the sterilizing unit.**

- **Make sure packaging material is appropriate for the method and device used.**

- **Never use staples, paper clips, or other sharp items to seal packaging as these can puncture the package.**

- **Do not use paper or plastic packaging material for more than one cycle of sterilization.**

- **Separate plastic and metal instruments prior to packaging. Metal instruments are good conductors of heat, and can potentially melt or distort plastic.**

- **Note variations in heat and pressure for different cycles, (i.e. packs and wraps) to prevent damage to sensitive instruments.**

- **Always perform routine maintenance on all sterilization equipment according to manufacturer's instructions and keep maintenance records.**

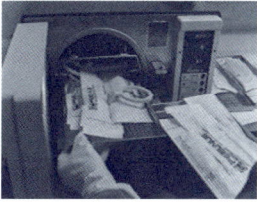

It is critical to your Exposure Control Program to ensure that complete sterilization occurs. However, you cannot tell that an instrument is truly sterilized simply by looking at it. In fact, there are a number of reasons sterilization may fail:

- **Improper equipment maintenance**
- **A damaged gasket or seal on the door of the sterilizer**
- **Improper cycle time**
- **Too many instruments in one package or too many packages for one cycle.** An improper load organization may prevent steam/heat circulation and penetration of the packages.
- **Inappropriate packaging material**
- **Inappropriate instruments or items for a particular sterilization method**
- **Multiple layers of packaging materials**

To routinely achieve sterilization of reprocessed items, remember to:

- **Use the tips above**
- **Be consistent in using the equipment**
- **Follow the manufacturer's directions and your practice's SOP**
- **Monitor the process with cycle indicators, chemical indicators, and biologic monitors on a routine basis.** The goal of monitoring is to assess all components of the sterilization process, which determines whether or not sterilization is routinely achieved.
- **Document the monitoring to ensure quality control**
- **Use a biologic indicator for every sterilizer load that contains an implantable device. Verify results before using the implantable device, whenever possible.**

Mechanical Monitoring

Each time you reprocess instruments in your sterilizer, there are simple measurements that must be monitored. The correct methods are found in the manufacturer's instructions and your SOPs. Cycle indicators are observable measurements and are used similar to a pre-flight check in an aircraft. The following is an example for an autoclave:

- **Solution** - **Adequate?**
- **Temperature** - **Reached?**
- **Pressure** - **Reached?**
- **Time** - **Set after temperature and pressure are reached.**
- **Other** - **Are there any other factors that must be monitored or followed for your sterilizer?**

Note:

Some sterilizers can show documentation (e.g., paper printouts, digital software, etc.) of the above information. This does not verify sterilization, but only that the sterilization parameters have been reached.

Chemical Indicators

Chemical indicators (CI) are defined by the Association for the Advancement of Medical Instrumentation (AAMI) as "…sterilization process monitoring devices designed to respond with a chemical or physical change to one or more of the physical conditions within the sterilizing chamber. CIs are often used to detect sterilizer malfunction/failures resulting from improper loading of the sterilizer, incorrect packaging, deficiencies of the sterilizing agent, or malfunction of the sterilizer itself."

The "pass" or color change of a CI does not mean that the item or items in the sterilizer load are sterile; it means that the parameter or parameters for sterilization that the CI was designed to measure have been reached. The use of CIs is only one component of an effective sterility assurance program. Chemical indicators should be used in conjunction with a biological indicator (spore test), physical monitors, a sterilizer preventative maintenance program, and accurate record keeping for each sterilization load.

CDC recommends that chemical indicators be used on the *inside* of every pack of instruments and on the outside when the internal indicator is not visible from the outside. Association for the Advancement of Medical Instrumentation (AAMI) standards recommend use on both the inside and outside of every pack.

Single parameter indicators measure one parameter of sterilization (e.g., heat). Multi-parameter indicators measure two or more parameters of sterilization (e.g., heat, time, etc.).

The AAMI Standards list six types of chemical indicators:

Type	Indications for Use
Type 1	Process indicator for use on the exterior of packages.
Type 2	For use in specific tests procedures, i.e. *Bowie-Dick type* test to check for proper air removal of pre-vacuum steam sterilizers.
Type 3	Single-variable indicator that reacts to one critical variable, i.e. time or temperature.
Type 4	Multi-variable indicator that reacts to 2 or more critical variables.
Type 5	Integrating indicator that reacts to all critical variables and is equal in performance to a biological indicator, but does not replace routine biologic monitoring.
Type 6	Emulating indicator that reacts to all critical variables for a specified sterilization cycle.

ANSI/AAMI ST79:2017 Comprehensive guide to steam sterilization and sterility assurance in health care facilities www.aami.org/productspublications/ProductDetail.aspx?ItemNumber=1383

Notes:

- Single-parameter indicators display color change after being exposed to heat.

- Multi-parameter indicators display color change after being exposed to heat over time.

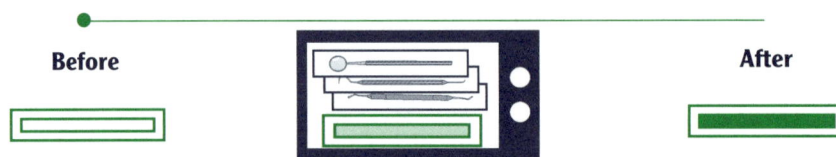

Before   After

All indicators must be specific to the sterilization method used. The following are ways of using process indicators:

1. **Place a chemical indicator inside each package of instruments** to identify that penetration of the sterilization agent through the packaging/wrapping material has occurred.

2. **If the internal indicator cannot be seen from the outside, use paper or paper/ plastic packaging material that has a rapid-change indicator as part of the package or place a strip outside packaging** to identify that a process has occurred.

3. **Use packaging tape with an indicator incorporated into it** to identify that a process has occurred.

Biologic Monitors

Biologic monitoring is the only method to verify sterilization. Biologic monitoring uses biologic indicators (BI) that are either paper strips, glass, or plastic vials containing non-pathogenic highly resistant bacterial endospores. When these strips or vials are processed through a successful sterilization cycle, the test dose of endospores is killed. There are two bacterial endospores used as biologic indicators: *Geobacillus stearothermopohilus* (for steam and unsaturated chemical vapor units) and *Bacillus atrophaeus* (for dry heat and ethylene oxide units).

Biologic Indicators, also called spore tests, are available as a mail-in-system where, after processing a paper strip BI along with a normal load, the BIs are sent to a lab for incubation. Test results are returned to the practice via phone, fax, mail or website.

Spore tests are also available as an in-office system where after processing a BI vial along with a normal load, the test BI and an *unprocessed* Control BI are incubated onsite. Always follow the specific manufacturer's instructions for these tests. Check the lot numbers; it is important that the control and test BIs come from the same spore lots. Note the test results in your records after full incubation of both BIs.

Always check the expiration dates on the spore strips for mail-in systems and the spore vials for the in-office systems. Expired spores will provide an invalid test with no growth on the test BI and no growth on the control BI.

Biologic Monitoring Time Schedule

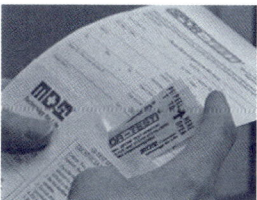

CDC recommends at least weekly biologic monitoring. Some states *require* that monitoring be done on either a weekly, monthly, or bi-monthly basis. Due to the importance of the information from the results of biologic monitoring, testing should be performed at least weekly. The type of equipment your practice uses, as well as the frequency of use, will help determine how often you perform biologic monitoring.

At a minimum you should biologically monitor:

· **One time per week**
· **The first cycle after repair of the unit, release the load only after a passing BI result. AAMI standards recommend 3 passed BI cycles before putting the sterilizer back into service.**
· **All implantable devices. This is not applicable in most dental settings; implants are delivered sterile by the manufacturer and should not be used if sterility is compromised.**
· **Initial use of a new sterilizer**
· **During training of new staff**
· **When a loading procedure is changed**
· **When processing hazardous waste on-site.**

To confirm sterilization, two BI strips or vials are used. A "test" BI is placed inside a test package of instruments and sterilized, and a "control" BI is held aside and not sterilized. When the sterilization cycle is complete, the test BI is removed from the test package, and both the test and control BIs are incubated for a specific amount of time.

Tips & Hints

- **Save several old or worn instruments to use as a test pack for biologic monitoring. Package these instruments and insert the test BI. After sterilizing and cooling, this package can be opened immediately without contaminating other instruments.**

Desired Results

The desired results are to have *no living endospores remaining* on the test BI, and to have endospore growth occurring on the control BI. If there are live spores on the test BI, sterilization did not occur and you must try to determine why and correct the problem. If there are no live spores on the control BI, the incubator did not work, or the initial control BI did not contain viable endospores.

Interpretation of Results

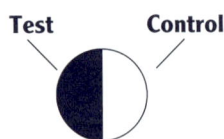

Test   Control

+ + **Sterilization NOT effective.**
Check sterilizer and carefully RE-DO TEST.

- + **DESIRED RESULT.**
Sterilization effective.

+ - **Sterilization NOT effective.**
Incubator may not be working, check incubator and sterilizer and carefully RE-DO TEST.

- - **No growth.**
Strips may have been old or expired, the incubator may not be functioning, or the control may have been mistakenly sterilized. Check & RE-DO TEST with new strips or vials.

If sterilization is not proven to be effective, i.e. a positive spore test, the following are recommended:

a. **Remove the sterilizer from service and review sterilization procedures (e.g., work practices and use of mechanical and chemical indicators) to determine whether operator error could be responsible.**

b. **Retest the sterilizer by using biologic, mechanical, and chemical indicators after correcting any identified procedural problems.**

c. **If the repeat spore test is negative, and mechanical and chemical indicators are within normal limits, put the sterilizer back in service.**

The following are recommended if the repeat spore test is positive:

a. **Do not use the sterilizer until it has been inspected or repaired or the exact reason for the positive test has been determined.**

b. **Recall, to the extent possible, and reprocess all items processed since the last negative spore test** (this is why you must keep careful records of your sterilization cycles).

c. **Before placing the sterilizer back in service, rechallenge the sterilizer with biologic indicator tests in three consecutive empty chamber sterilization cycles after the cause of the sterilizer failure has been determined and corrected.**

Facilities with large steam sterilizers should use a commercial test pack referred to as a *process challenge device* (PCD) to monitor their sterilizers—preferably with every load. The PCD is placed flat on the lowest shelf above the sterilizer drain.

PCD commercial test packs are available with a Type 5 or a Type 6 chemical indicator. These are used in each sterilization load. They can also be used with a biologic monitor (BI) for weekly or daily monitoring of steam sterilizers. No commercial PCD is available for chemical-vapor or dry heat sterilizers.

Use of a PCD in Dental Offices

Dental offices commonly release instruments for use before the results of the BI are known. If there is a BI failure, it is likely that suspect instruments have been used on patients subsequent to the sterilization failure. Monitoring each load with a PCD may avoid release of improperly or incompletely sterilized items because the chemical and mechanical test results are immediately available. A PCD can consist of a Type 5 integrating indicator contained in packaging that is the same or more challenging than the normal sterilization load contents.

PCD Configuration and Placement

Place a Type 5 integrating indicator in the geometric center of a test pack consisting of a wrapped cassette or tray, or the center of a test pouch of instruments. A PCD can also be made by placing a Type 5 integrating indicator inside 3 layers of sterilization wrap and folding the layers of wrap to create 9 layers around the Type 5 integrating indicator.

The test pack should be placed in the center of a load. Upon removal of the load, check the indicator before releasing the load. The use of a PCD does not eliminate the need to include a chemical indicator (CI) inside each pack of instruments.

Note:

Monitoring sterilization is a complicated process. For this reason, many dental practices have the endospore incubation done by an independent laboratory that provides the strips/vials and keeps all the necessary records. If the process is performed in-house, you should still use an outside service to check your own results on a periodic basis. For any monitoring performed by an outside service, be sure to receive duplicate records for your own practice's files.

Considerations for Dental Handpieces

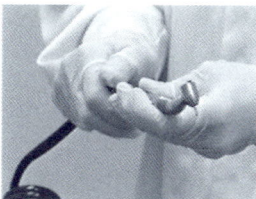

Dental handpieces require special considerations for reprocessing:

- **They contact oral tissue and fluids.**
- **They contain a number of irregular, rough surfaces that make cleaning difficult.**
- **They draw (suck back) saliva and potentially blood into their inner components.**

The CDC recommends that handpieces that can be removed from the air and water lines of the dental unit be sterilized between patients and a sterile handpiece be used for each patient, according to the specific handpiece manufacturer's directions for reprocessing. Scientific evidence has demonstrated contamination of the internal components including the motor of both high and slow speed handpieces that are removed from air and waterlines of the dental unit. These recommendations include:

1. **Clean and heat-sterilize handpieces and other intraoral instruments that can be removed from the air and waterlines of dental units between patients.**
2. **Follow the manufacturer's instructions for cleaning, lubrication, and sterilization of handpieces and other intraoral instruments that can be removed from the air and waterlines of dental units.**
3. **Do not surface-disinfect, use liquid chemical sterilants or ethylene oxide on handpieces and other intraoral instruments that can be removed from the air and waterlines of dental units.**

The FDA in its March 1993 "FDA Medical Bulletin" included a section on the sterilization of dental handpieces:

"FDA recommends that reusable dental drill handpieces and related instruments (such as air or water syringes and ultrasonic scalers) be heat-sterilized between patients to reduce the risk of disease transmission.

If a handpiece cannot withstand heat sterilization, it should be retrofitted to increase heat tolerance and then sterilized. If this can't be done, the handpiece should no longer be used. Chemical disinfection is not recommended.

Although no documented cases of disease transmission have been associated with contaminated dental handpieces, the ADA also recommends sterilization of these instruments between patients. The CDC also recommends that dental handpieces be autoclaved or replaced if they are not currently heat-stable."

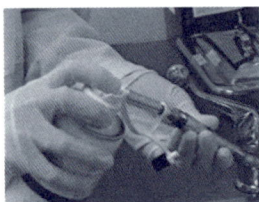

Always follow the specific manufacturer instructions for sterilization and maintenance of dental handpieces. As when cleaning other instruments, proper PPE should be worn and Standard Precautions should be followed. Handpieces must be cleaned to remove external debris before packaging for sterilization. This can be accomplished using a sponge with mild soap and water or water alone. One difference between handpieces and other instruments, however, is the need for lubrication (which may affect the packaging of handpieces). Some manufacturers recommend lubrication before sterilization, others require it both before and after, and some handpieces are "lube-free."

There are also dental handpieces that are independent of the air and waterlines. CDC recommends you follow the specific manufacturer's directions for reprocessing.

Handpiece Sterilization/Asepsis Procedures

Using the manufacturer's instructions for your practice's handpieces, fill out the table below.

- **Enter the brand name and model number (name) of each handpiece in use.**
- **Consult the manufacturer's instructions for the parameters for sterilization.**
- **Use a different row for each handpiece, such as high speed, low speed, fiber-optic, etc.** (Extra space is provided in the event your practice adds or replaces handpieces in the future).

BRAND/Model	ULTRASONIC CLEANING	CLEAN/LUBE TYPE	LUBRICATION TIME	MAX. TEMP.	METHOD OF STERILIZATION
List Brand/ Model #	YES or NO	Spray, Drop Oil, Other	Before and/or After Sterilization	in °F or °C	Type

Discussion

Discuss with your Infection Control Coordinator or Safety Officer the specific standard operating procedures for reprocessing instruments and reusable patient care items.

Notes

Objectives

Upon completion of this course on product selection, you will be able to:

1. Describe some products used in dentistry that fall under the jurisdiction of:
   - U.S. Food and Drug Administration (FDA)
   - U.S. Environmental Protection Agency (EPA)

2. Identify criteria that should be considered before making a purchasing decision.

3. List three general categories of cleaning agents.

4. Explain selection criteria for environmental surface disinfectants in dental healthcare settings.

5. Explain criteria to be considered when selecting Personal Protective Equipment (PPE) for purchase.

6. Explain the significance of the tuberculocidal claim for hospital disinfectants.

7. Describe key factors for choosing disinfection chemicals.

Focus

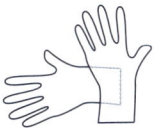

Product selection is a key component of any program, yet there is no one perfect product for any given procedure or task. There is, however, a best product for a specific practice or provider. Development of a site-specific framework for the cost effective selection and use of infection control products is essential for a well-managed practice.

Your Role in Purchasing

What is your role in purchasing? Although a detailed analysis of products may be made by the person in charge of purchasing, your input is critical. Do you feel one product works or fits your practice better than another? Why? Are there any chemicals to which you are allergic? Is there certain equipment in your office which hinders your ability to follow the practices of effective exposure control? These concerns should be communicated to your Infection Control Coordinator or Safety Officer to improve product selection for your office.

Your Role in Inventory Control

An additional role for everyone in the office is inventory control. Inventory control is the process of ordering, rotating, storing, using, disposing, and the subsequent reordering of equipment and supplies. For example, you may open the last box of gloves in your size or you may discover that a chemical in inventory is near or past its expiration date. It is your responsibility to inform the appropriate person of any new status or problems with inventory, so replacements can be ordered.

Product Information

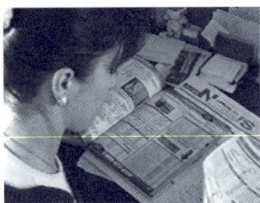

Detailed information about dental products is essential to make informed choices. This information comes from a variety of places:

- **Professional journals and scientific literature** provide research-based scientific information on the safety and efficacy of the active ingredients of products.

- **Sales people** should be able to provide technical data and answer questions about the products they sell. Their expertise may be limited to their product line and they may or may not be knowledgeable on products offered by competitors.

- **Catalogs** may be a convenient method of purchasing products. They may not provide enough in-depth information, particularly when you are purchasing a product for the first time.

- **Dental trade magazines** may review products in articles, which can give you information concerning the effectiveness of products or how certain products compare with one another.

- **Trade shows, internet web sites and manufacturer's representatives** are a way to get information directly from manufacturers and distributors. Again, you may or may not be provided with information about competing products.

- **Product comparisons,** if done properly, may be your best source for product evaluation. The best sources for reports on these evaluations are in the peer-reviewed literature.

- **Colleagues** may be able to offer valuable information from a current user's perspective.

Product Guarantees

No matter what the claims of a salesperson or catalog, it is ultimately the responsibility of the manufacturer to guarantee the performance and safety of its products. You must, however, use products according to manufacturer's directions.

Government Regulations

Prior to purchasing chemicals, dental materials, or medical devices, be aware that these products come under the jurisdiction of the EPA, the FDA, or both:

EPA: Registers all chemicals, disinfectants, and decontaminants that impact the environment, under FIFRA: the Federal Insecticide, Fungicide, and Rodenticide Act. Products registered with the EPA will have a registration number on the label.

FDA: Has jurisdiction over medical devices and accessories to medical devices, food, and drugs. Manufacturers must provide safety and efficacy data to receive market clearance by the FDA. Examples of medical devices in dentistry include ultrasonic cleaners, radiographic equipment, sterilization equipment, chemical products that make sterilant claims, and gloves.

Purchasing Analysis

There is no single answer to any purchasing decision. Regardless of the product, there are several criteria you should consider to ensure that the product is the right one for the job, acceptable to staff and patients, and cost effective. This analysis is part of any purchasing decision.

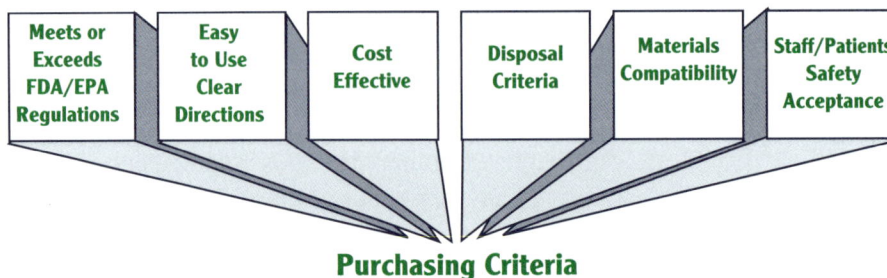

Meets or Exceeds FDA/EPA Regulations	Easy to Use Clear Directions	Cost Effective	Disposal Criteria	Materials Compatibility	Staff/Patients Safety Acceptance

Purchasing Criteria

Chemical agents used in dentistry generally fall into three categories: cleaning agents, surface disinfectants, and immersion disinfectants. *Cleaning agents* may be any surfactant used to clean environmental surfaces. A *surface* disinfectant is used to decontaminate environmental surfaces, as covered in Course #4, while *immersion* disinfectants are used to decontaminate certain types of reusable semi-critical items that cannot withstand any other available sterilization process.

Several questions should be asked when purchasing a product:

- **What are the use claims for the chemical? Is it a surface-only or an immersion disinfectant?**
- **Does it have the proper regulatory clearance?**
- **Does a certain temperature affect the disinfection time?**
- **Are there any special precautions to observe when using the chemical?**
- **How is it safely disposed?**
- **What is its shelf life, use life, and, for immersion chemicals, reuse life?**
- **Is it easily deactivated by debris or bioburden?**
- **Is it compatible with the materials, surfaces, and other equipment on which it is used?**
- **Does anyone in the office have allergies or sensitivities to a particular chemical or a component used in the chemical?**

Chemical Labels

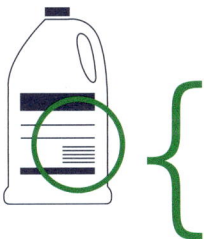

Just as you read food labels at the supermarket to find product ingredients, nutritional values and expiration dates, you must also read labels on the chemical products prior to use. Labels must contain the following information:

- **Active ingredient(s)**
- **Precautionary information**
- **Disposal instructions**
- **Use life and/or reuse life**
- **Directions for use**
- **EPA registration number**
- **Expiration date, or shelf life**
- **Manufacturer name and address**

The label is a primary source of information for the proper use of a chemical, but you should check manufacturer's directions and the product's Safety Data Sheet (SDS) for complete information. The active ingredients and precautionary information will help you know what PPE are necessary when using the product. The expiration date, or shelf life, indicates how long the product can be stored, while use life refers to how long the agent works once a product has been prepared for use (activated and/or diluted). Reuse life indicates both duration and the number of times an immersion chemical solution can be used for immersion disinfection or sterilization.

Disinfectants

Antimicrobial products are classified into three levels: sanitizer, disinfectant, and high-level disinfectant/sterilant. Disinfectants are further categorized into three levels, referred to by CDC as: low, intermediate, and high. In dentistry, intermediate-level disinfectants are used to disinfect noncritical surfaces, while high-level immersion chemicals are used to disinfect semicritical items that cannot withstand heat or ethylene oxide sterilization.

High-Level Disinfectants

- **Immersion high-level disinfection or immersion sterilization**
- **These disinfectants have the ability to kill bacterial endospores, *Mycobacterium tuberculosis*, hydrophilic and lipophilic viruses, fungi, and vegetative bacteria when used according to directions for high-level immersion disinfection.**
- **Glutaraldehydes, hydrogen peroxide, paracetic acid**
- **Note:** These cannot be biologic monitored so you can only assume sterilization occurs if the conditions are met.

Intermediate-Level Disinfectants

- **Used for clinical contact surfaces, especially those contaminated with blood**
- **Disinfects only**
- **Destroys *Mycobacterium tuberculosis*, hydrophilic and lipophilic viruses, fungi, and vegetative bacteria**
- **Iodophors, alcohol, synthetic phenolics, dual or synergized quaternaries, containing alcohol, sodium bromide, and chlorine**

Low-Level Disinfectants

- **Used for general housekeeping and clinical contact surfaces that are not contaminated with blood**
- **Destroys certain viruses and fungi, but not *Mycobacterium tuberculosis***
- **Simple quaternary ammonium compounds, detergents**

EPA-Registered Disinfectants

The Environmental Protection Agency (EPA) registers three types of disinfectants: limited, broad-spectrum and hospital. An EPA-registered hospital disinfectant is a broad-spectrum disinfectant that is also effective against some bacteria and viruses. An EPA-registered hospital disinfectant falls under the CDC category of a low-level disinfectant. When an EPA-registered hospital disinfectant also has a tuberculocidal claim, it is effective against even more bacteria and viruses including tuberculosis (TB), and falls under the CDC category of an intermediate-level disinfectant.

Resistance of Microorganisms to Germicidal Chemicals

The choice of specific cleaning or disinfecting agents is largely a matter of judgement, guided by product label claims and instructions and government regulations. A single liquid chemical germicide might not satisfy all disinfection requirements in a given dental practice or facility. Realistic use of liquid chemical germicides depends on consideration of multiple factors, including the degree of microbial killing required; the nature and composition of the surface, item, or device to be treated; and the cost, safety, and ease of use of the available agents. Selecting one appropriate product with a higher degree of potency to cover all situations might be more convenient.

Organism	Processing Level Required

Sterilization

Bacterial spores ———————————————— **FDA sterilant/high level disinfectant**
Geobacillus stearothermophilus **(= CDC sterilant/high-level disinfectant)**
Bacillus atrophaeus

Mycobacteria ———————— **EPA hospital disinfectant with**
Mycobacterium tuberculosis **tuberculocidal claim**
(= CDC intermediate-level disinfectant)

Nonlipid or small viruses
Polio virus
Coxsackle virus
Rhinovirus

Fungi
Aspergillus
Candida

Vegetative bacteria ———— **EPA hospital disinfectant**
Staphylococcus species **(= CDC low-level disinfectant)**
Pseudomonus species
Salmonella species

Lipid or medium-sized viruses
Human immunodeficiency virus
Herpes simplex virus
Hepatitis B and hepatitis C
Coronavirus

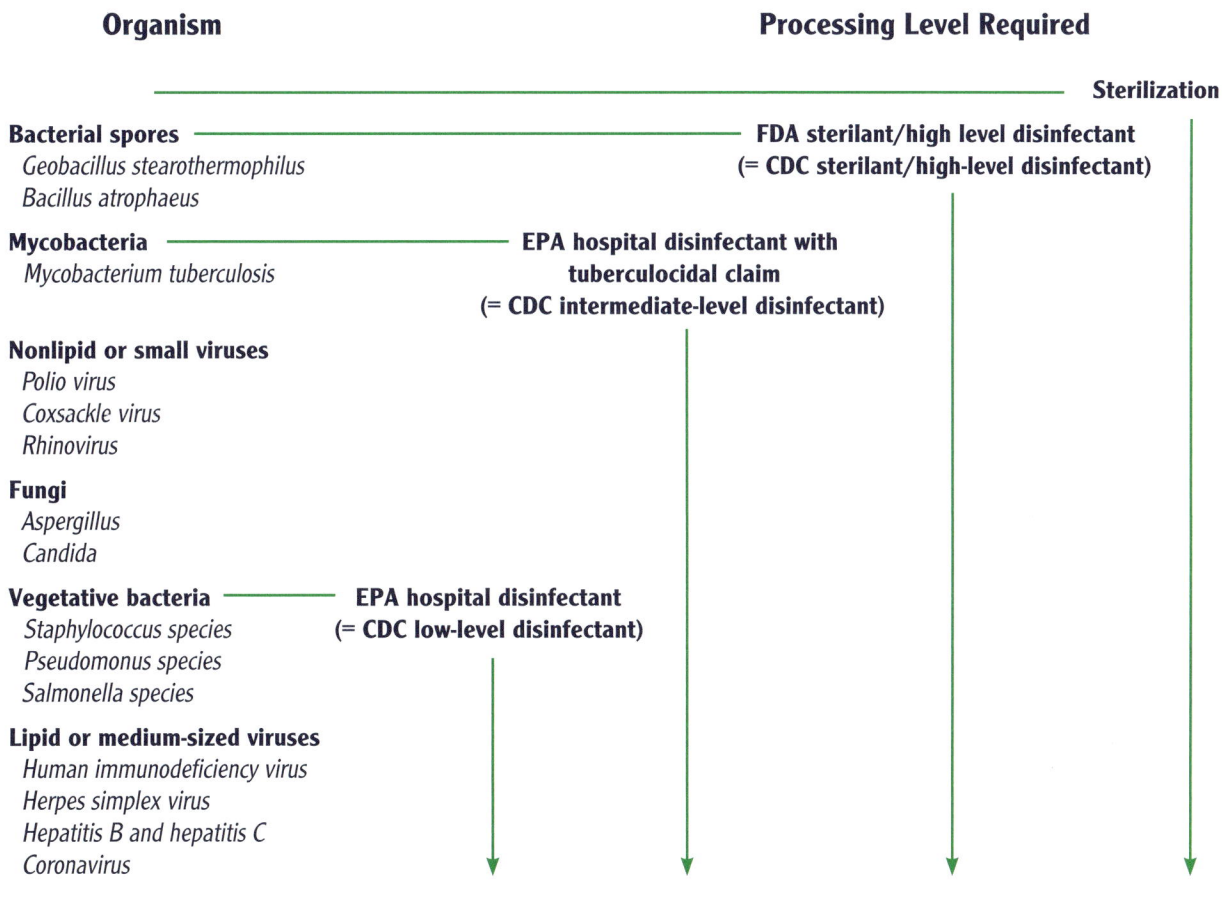

Source: Adapted from "Guidelines for Infection Control in Dental Health-Care Settings, 2003," MMWR, Dec. 19, 2003, Vol. 52, No. RR-17.

Surface Disinfectants

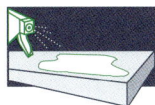

Intermediate-level surface disinfectants are used on environmental surfaces that become contaminated during patient care (clinical contact surfaces). This includes surfaces that are touched with contaminated gloved hands, are at risk for spatter contamination, or that come in contact with contaminated dental materials and instruments. Disinfectants should only be used on smooth hard surfaces. Non-smooth hard surfaces, such as grooved, ribbed areas or connections such as switches, are more effectively protected using surface covers (environmental barriers).

No one product is going to specifically meet all of your needs. When making purchasing decisions, you should choose a surface disinfectant that, at a minimum, answers the following questions:

1. **Does it meet the standards for an intermediate-level surface chemical?**

2. **Is it compatible with the surfaces on which it is being used and with the people using the chemical?**

3. **Is it easy to use? Are the directions understandable? Is it clearly marked? Is the contact time to kill *Mycobacterium tuberculosis* realistic for your practice?**

All disinfectants should be selected with the goal of achieving the highest level of disinfection possible. In the case of surface disinfectants, the label must indicate the amount of time required to kill *Mycobacterium tuberculosis* (TB). Other microorganisms are not as resistant as *M. tuberculosis*, so by eliminating the TB bacteria, you effectively reduce a large number of other less resistant bacteria, fungi and viruses, including HIV and HBV. Always check the kill claim and contact time for tuberculocidal action when more than one kill claim exists. To determine if a product meets these standards, look for any of these phrases on the label:

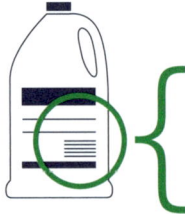

- **Tuberculocidal**

- **Intermediate-level surface disinfectant**

- **Hospital-level disinfectant**

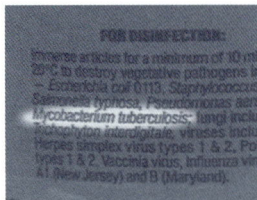

Any of these claims, combined with an EPA registration number, mean the product has completed minimum scientific testing to be registered as a surface disinfectant. If a product does not carry one of these claims, it may not be an appropriate surface disinfectant for a medical/dental environment. Or, if a product takes longer than 10 minutes to kill *Mycobacterium tuberculosis* at room temperature, do not consider it for use, since this is not a practical time-frame for operatory processing.

Surface Compatibility:

Once you have determined that an environmental surface disinfectant meets the standards necessary, you should consider its compatibility with surfaces and the people using the product. No disinfectant is perfect. They all have some drawbacks and part of the purchasing process is deciding which one has the greatest number of benefits with the least disadvantages for your practice.

Notes:

- Surfaces must be cleaned prior to disinfection.
- Research indicates that water-based disinfectants have surfactant qualities and can effectively clean a surface as well as disinfect it. This requires the use of the product in two separate steps: cleaning, followed by disinfection, as discussed in Course #4.

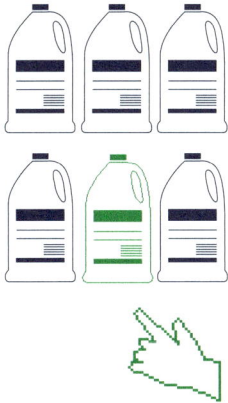

SURFACE (Intermediate-Level)

- **EPA Registration number**
- **Tuberculocidal**
- **Shelf Life, Use Life**
- **Concentration (activation)**
- **Temperature/Time**
- **Use: Full Strength or Diluted**
- **Warnings: Disposal, Toxic Effects, Precautions**
- **Limitations**
- **Storage and Disposal Requirements**
- **Hard Water Effectiveness** (Note: hard water reduces the effectiveness of some products, especially iodophors)
- **Manufacturer's Directions and Registered claims**
- **NOTE: THE MOST IMPORTANT STEP IS ADEQUATE CLEANING -** Check to see if chemical can be used as a cleaner.

IMMERSION (High-Level)

Except for the EPA registration number, all items under Surface Disinfectants plus:

- **Sporicidal**
- **Shelf Life, Use and Reuse Life**
- **Concentration/Activation**
- **Time and Temperature Required for Immersion Disinfection**
- **Time and Temperature Required for Immersion Sterilization**
- **FDA Clearance to Market as an Immersion High-Level Disinfectant/ Sterilant**
  - will not appear on label
  - check with distributor for FDA clearance information

Staff/Patient Compatibility:

All chemicals used should be as nontoxic as possible to prevent potential respiratory or dermal (skin) hazards. Staff or patients, however, may have specific allergies or sensitivities to certain chemicals, which would prohibit or restrict their use. An example is iodophor, one of the oldest generic disinfectants, which is registered as an effective tuberculocidal surface disinfectant. If a staff member or patient is sensitive to iodine, a different, noniodine chemical may be a safer choice. Most iodine sensitivities are to ingested iodine; contact or environmental exposure is usually not a problem. This should be determined on a case-by-case basis, in consultation with a physician.

The final purchasing considerations are user satisfaction and cost. User satisfaction takes into account the storage, mixture, use, and disposal of a product, while cost considerations compare equivalent products in an effort to minimize expenditures while maintaining safety and efficiency.

- Must the chemical be stored and/or used within a certain temperature range?
- What PPE, other safety equipment, or simple items such as a funnel, are needed?
- Some disinfectant chemicals come in concentrated form. The directions should include full-strength use or dilution ratio for mixing the concentrate with water.
- If the chemical is to be diluted with water, is tap water acceptable? Some chemicals may be affected by a high mineral content in tap water, which will reduce the effectiveness of a disinfectant and require you to use distilled water.
- Who will be responsible for diluting or mixing disinfectants?
- What is the use life of the diluted disinfectant? If it is not mixed fresh daily, is there an indicator to determine when the dilution use life has expired?

For disinfectants that are sprayed on a surface, consider nonaerosol spray, pump-type bottles. For concentrated chemicals that must be diluted, does the manufacturer provide bottles that come appropriately labeled – including hazard communication information? If not, you must purchase pump bottles and label them with the hazard communication information yourself.

Disposal Considerations

Finally, how easy is it to discard the chemical? You can dispose of most nonhazardous chemical disinfectants down the drain with plenty of water. There may be, however, state and local restrictions on disposal, or special considerations for septic systems. (Course #9)

Note:

Some disposal directions indicate that "copious" amounts of water are necessary for disposal down "household" drains. Copious water requires at least a 30-to-1 ratio, or 1 gallon of chemical requires 30 gallons of water to dispose of properly. This may also depend on the type of sewage or septic system in use at your facility.

If the chemical is able to be disposed down the drain and has a surfactant, you may instead wish to run any remaining solution through your dental suction lines. This serves multiple purposes by decontaminating and cleaning the suction lines, eliminating the need for a separate product for suction cleaning, and reducing the waste. The manufacturer of the chemical product and the suction equipment manufacturer should be contacted prior to using the product in this manner.

If a chemical is labeled as "hazardous," there will be specific manufacturer's instructions for disposal on the product label and the SDS. Additional information should be in your Infection Control/Exposure Control Plan, which reflects federal, state, and local hazardous waste regulations.

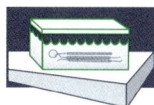

Immersion disinfectants are primarily used for high-level disinfection/sterilization of reusable semi-critical items that cannot withstand heat or ethylene oxide exposure. Manufacturer's instructions must be followed to achieve the conditions for sterilization or disinfection. For example, if the manufacturer indicates that instruments must be immersed undisturbed for 10 hours, then sterilization cannot be assumed if they are removed after two hours. An additional complication is that immersion chemicals cannot be biologic monitored, so sterilization cannot be verified. Indicators should be used to ensure the minimum effective concentration of the chemical and at no time should a chemical be used past its expiration date.

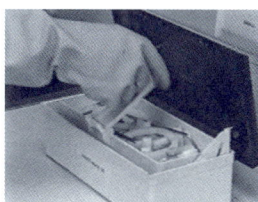

Immersion disinfectants are considered medical devices by the FDA and therefore need to be cleared for marketing by this agency. Many of the same issues apply when purchasing immersion or surface disinfectants. The product must be easy to use, as nontoxic as possible to employees, and meet specific FDA requirements. Since most of these chemicals are hazardous, extra care needs to be taken regarding handling, storage, use, and disposal.

If you have any questions regarding any chemical, it is best to call or write the manufacturer for specific chemical information or consult the EPA or FDA for generic information.

If you use Immersion Disinfectants, how long should the items be immersed to meet the conditions for sterilization?
(Hint: See the label of the product used in your practice)

_____

_____

_____

Equipment

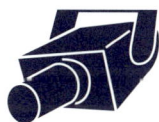

Many of the same general considerations made when purchasing chemicals also apply to buying supplies and equipment. *Supplies* are "disposable equipment" and include items such as gloves or other PPE. These are purchased frequently, while *equipment* such as instruments, sterilizers, unit chairs, etc., are replaced far less frequently.

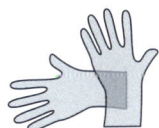

Careful attention must be paid to manufacturers' instructions for use, maintenance, and/or disposal. This is to ensure that the product or equipment is used in a safe and effective manner. These directions or instructions are included with the product literature and should describe the specific use, care, and limitations of a given product. For example, handpieces may or may not need lubrication; autoclaves may require distilled water; immersion disinfectants should not be used in an ultrasonic cleaner; a toaster oven should not be used as a sterilizer (the instructions only say how to heat food); or... the list goes on and on. You should take the time to become familiar with the literature provided when you buy equipment to ensure proper use. As with chemicals, equipment must be used according to the manufacturer's instructions.

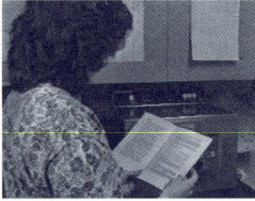

Much of the equipment used in dentistry is considered to be "medical devices" or "accessories to medical devices" and consequently come under the jurisdiction of the FDA. Medical devices include sterilizers, radiographic equipment, gloves, as well as other equipment you use, and must therefore, receive "clearance for market" by the FDA. In addition to ensuring that medical devices meet safety and efficacy specifications, the FDA stipulates that any safety problems associated with products or equipment and reported to a manufacturer must, in turn, be reported by the manufacturer to the FDA. It is to your benefit to report any problems you have to the manufacturer and possibly to the FDA as well. If there are ongoing identifiable problems with a medical device, the FDA may take action.

Note:

If you experience problems with a medical device, you should first contact the manufacturer, then, if the problem persists, contact the FDA. If a device-related injury occurs, then report it to the FDA MedWatch program 1-800-FDA-1088 or visit the FDA website at www.fda.gov for more information.

Personal Protective Equipment (PPE)

PPE is one of the primary focuses in exposure control, and therefore careful attention must be made to its selection. PPE includes gloves, eyewear, face masks, face shields, and garments. PPE are considered "medical devices" and are regulated by the FDA.

Many of the considerations for PPE were covered in Course #3 and should be reviewed when making purchasing decisions. For example, with patient treatment gloves, you must consider:

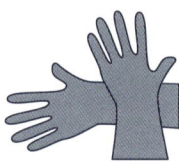

- **Shelf life**
- **Fit**
- **Material: Latex, vinyl, nitrile, neoprene, other synthetics**
- **Potential allergies/sensitivities of staff and patients**
- **Limitations for specific use**
- **Specific tasks that require specific types of gloves**
- **Sterile or nonsterile**

Special Considerations for Latex Gloves:

- **Purchase only powder-free latex gloves (powered gloves have been banned by the FDA).**
- **Examine the shipments of nonsterile gloves for dampness or water stains.
  As with any damaged shipments, they should not be accepted.**
- **Check for dampness or mold on glove dispensing boxes and each glove before using.
  Signs of mold include a musty odor, discoloration, or small black spots.**
- **Use only surgeon's gloves for surgical procedures.**

Consider both the filtration effectiveness and the fit for face masks. Select eyewear that meets the standards of protective eyewear, e.g., high-impact lenses and solid side shields. To protect the arms, neck, and upper body, gowns should be fluid resistant and of a style to protect the skin and clothing at risk of potential aerosol and spatter exposure (long-sleeved, high-neck, knee-length). If gowns are going to be reused, they must be machine washable in hot water and able to withstand heat drying.

Barrier Surface Covers

As covered in Course #4, the use of disposable barriers provides protection to underlying equipment and surfaces, and facilitates easy changes between patients. Barriers are manufactured to specifically fit specialized equipment and surfaces and are available in generic shapes and sizes. Additionally, the most common materials are fluid-proof plastic and fluid-proof plastic-backed paper.

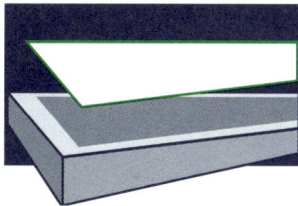

Plastic-backed Paper Barrier on Countertop

Plastic Bag over Ribbed Hose

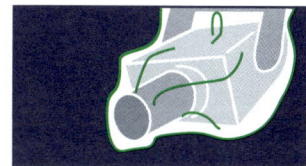

Custom-Designed Barrier for X-Ray Tube Head

The surface that will be protected will determine which type of barrier(s) should be used. As indicated in Course #4, plastic-backed paper works well on flat surfaces such as instrument trays or countertops, but with some equipment, such as ribbed hoses, only plastic surface barriers will conform to the surface. The barrier on an FDA cleared medical device must also be FDA cleared.

Fitted barriers may, at first glance, be more expensive than a simple alternative such as barrier wrap. However, the added time needed to cut, apply and remove the barrier wrap, may make plastic surface barriers more cost effective.

Tips & Hints

- **Colored barriers may increase compliance and prevent contamination as they provide a visual cue of what can be touched.**

Major Equipment Purchases

Unlike PPE and barrier protectors, major equipment such as sterilizing equipment, ultrasonic cleaners, thermal disinfectors, dental units, X-ray units, and other equipment are purchased much less frequently. Analysis is crucial to ensure a successful purchase, as equipment must suit the specific needs of your practice. With sterilizers, for example, it may be more cost effective to use two different types of sterilizers. This takes into account the sterilizing limitations of various instruments, handpieces, and other items, and allows you to sterilize a greater number of instruments simultaneously.

Major equipment may influence other purchasing issues. For example, the choice of a specific type of sterilizer will, in turn, require that specific types of packaging material be used (Course #5). In addition, if your practice is moving to instrument cassettes, you must make sure that the cassettes will properly fit into your present sterilizers and ultrasonic cleaners. It may be necessary to purchase new equipment or choose other models.

List the sterilizers in your practice and the appropriate packaging for each.

Sterilizer: _____

Packaging: _____

Sterilizer: _____

Packaging: _____

As your practice updates and replaces major pieces of equipment, such as dental chairs or radiographic equipment, you need to consider exposure control features in deciding what to purchase.

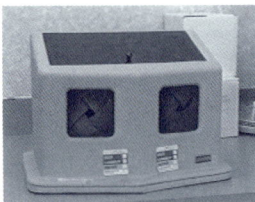

- **Equipment purchased should be "exposure control friendly," to allow for efficient and effective cleaning and disinfecting or cleaning and barrier-protecting.**
- **Furniture should be streamlined and smooth, to facilitate cleaning. If renovating the operatory, you should replace carpeting with vinyl flooring.**
- **Cabinets, shelving, and counters must have a chip-resistant finish. The use of wood, fabric, and plants in operatories should be avoided, as they are difficult to decontaminate.**
- **If you use patient education materials during treatment, they should be laminated for easy decontamination.**

In general, you are striving for an operatory that is as easy to clean as possible, which will both streamline operatory processing and provide your patients with the assurance that the treatment area is safe.

Cost

Cost is always an important consideration when selecting equipment and products, however it is critical to look beyond the invoice price as other factors may contribute to the bottom line or true cost.

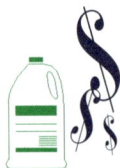

In determining true product cost, you should conduct an analysis that considers other factors in addition to the actual purchase price. The initial cost of a product considers only the purchase price, while the true cost takes into account any hidden costs or benefits that may exist. For example, an analysis may show that a product that is the least expensive initially may be more costly over a period of time. This may be due to the need for more frequent replacements or additional employee time necessary to use properly.

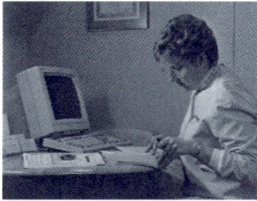

Suppose a salesperson suggests you buy cassettes for instruments to simplify reprocessing and storage as well as to protect both instruments and staff. Your first thought may be that cassettes are a costly alternative to your present method. But making a cost-effective decision means you should consider any extra costs *and* savings.

- **Cassettes are reusable and stack easily for storage. All storage areas must be clean and dry, but cassettes may necessitate additional or reorganized storage areas.**
- **Instruments are tightly secured within the cassette, ensuring less damage to instruments during processing, which reduces total instrument cost through less frequent replacements.**
- **Clinicians handle contaminated instruments less frequently, reducing the potential for sharps injuries and related costs of managing an injury.**
- **Cassettes may speed up processing time through reduced instrument handling.**
- **Cassettes may require related supportive equipment and supplies such as size-compatible ultrasonic cleaners, sterilizers, and package wrapping.**

Taking into account the above considerations, you can complete a cost comparison for the potential practice life of the equipment.

Cost Comparison Example

SAVINGS/COST for Expected Life	PRESENT METHOD vs. CASSETTES
· Initial Cassette Cost	· $/Cassettes (Initial Cost)
· Instrument Replacement Cost	· Expected Savings over Historical Expenditures
· Additional Equipment Costs	· New Sterilizer and/or Ultrasonic Cleaner?
· Employee Time: Processing	· Expected Savings over 1st Year
· Employee Time: Operatory Set-up	· Expected Savings over 1st Year
· Packaging Expenses	· New Barrier Wraps vs. Old Packaging
· Other?	
Actual Cost	**Savings or Increased Cost of Cassettes**

This does not take into account benefits such as increased value of patient and staff safety. As an example of assigning value to these benefits, you may want to consider the cost of managing an Exposure Incident, including the cost of medical follow-up.

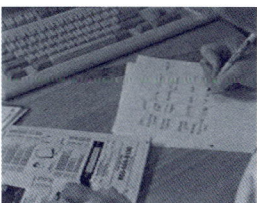

The actual cost in the previous example will be different for each practice. Practices that have an efficient system for reprocessing instruments, or those that are tight on space, may find their present system satisfactory or less expensive. Others may find cassettes more efficient and a cost savings. You should always do your own analysis, using information from all sources. Do not rely exclusively on any one source, including salespeople, manufacturer's reps, or even the example above.

Price Comparison

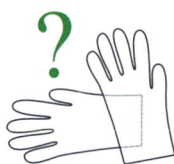

Another example of cost analysis is to compare two similar products. Burs for handpieces come in many varieties and prices. However, because they are made of carbon steel, they may corrode or become dull when sterilized in steam autoclaves. The alternative would be to purchase less expensive single-use disposable burs. Another variable in your analysis would be to purchase an additional sterilizer, such as a dry heat sterilizer, for carbon steel instruments.

Other Purchasing Considerations

Some products are available in large quantities at a lower unit cost. You may decide to buy gloves or a chemical in bulk, but you must consider the shelf life of the product and available storage space.

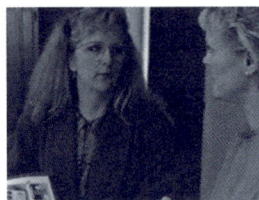

Storage space can have a direct effect on your purchasing decisions. As an example, using vinyl gloves for nonpatient treatment tasks that do not require puncture-resistant gloves is prudent because they are less expensive and reduce latex exposure. Some practices may not stock vinyl gloves due to space limitations and, instead, rely on latex gloves for all procedures that do not require puncture-resistant utility gloves. In addition, there may be staff preferences for gloves, adding another element to the purchasing decision.

Basically all dental practices must balance the cost of a product against its effectiveness. In choosing products, you must take into account:

- **How the product is used**
- **How often you use it**
- **How it is packaged**
- **Storage requirements and shelf life**
- **Staff and patient Safety**
- **Staff preferences, needs, and sensitivities**
- **The quality and reliability of sales support by the manufacturer and/or distributor**

Summary

Proper analysis will determine the best product, brand of product, vendor, and quantity to be ordered. The challenge is to remain open to new technology and products, and to use sound judgement and cost-effective decision making in the selection and purchasing process.

Your personal role as a consumer of dental products is an important one, and as a user, you can provide valuable information for your practice. You should inform your Infection Control Coordinator or Safety Officer of your observations, preferences and difficulties with any existing products or new products that may save the practice time or money and make your job safer and easier.

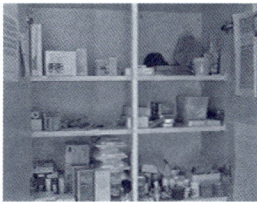

The organization and control of inventory focuses on the rotation and best use of supplies. These aspects of inventory control relate to purchasing, as the need for a steady supply of chemicals and equipment must be balanced with both the need to ensure that items are used before their expiration date and the availability of storage space.

When and how often do you order various products? The initial order of supplies and equipment will be based on an assessment of use and storage capacity. Obviously, if your storage area is small, you will have to reorder more frequently. Your Infection Control Coordinator or Safety Officer will be able to tell you who does the ordering in your office, as well as how often supplies are ordered.

Stock Shortages

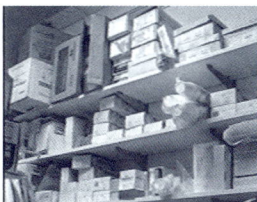

How often have you gone to get something and found a box or a shelf empty? As you use items, you must inform the person doing the ordering if an item needs to be replaced. All practices use an ordering system and the more established a system is, the easier it is for staff to assist in the process. Ordering systems can range from simple index cards, to bar code readers, to sophisticated computer-based systems. Some distributors can supply inventory/ordering systems that may make inventory organization and control more efficient. For any system, the following information may be useful:

- **Exact product name and manufacturer's/distributor's product number**
- **Where the item is stored**
- **Last order date**
- **Quantity ordered and price**
- **Reorder point**

Rotate Stock

As new supplies are received, you must remember to pull the older items from the back of storage areas and replace with the newer stock. This will ensure that previously purchased supplies don't remain in the back of cabinets and drawers and become outdated.

Tips & Hints

- **Before you place a large order to purchase a new item, get a sample, test it in the office, and get everyone's opinion. This can save money on purchases that don't meet your expectations.**

Discussion

Discuss with your Infection Control Coordinator or Safety Officer the specific standard operating procedures for inventory control and any role you may have in ordering supplies and equipment.

Notes

Objectives

Upon completion of this course on written procedures, you will be able to:

1. Identify within your Infection Control/Exposure Control Plan, one example of each:
   - Procedures
   - Records
   - Documentation

2. Explain the role of the Employee Health Record.

3. Briefly describe the use of a chemical inventory.

4. List three or more areas to be considered when performing a hazard audit.

Focus

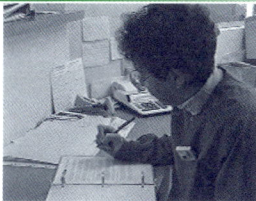

From chemical inventories, to waste disposal manifests, to your own personal health record, written reports are used to prevent accidents, help in emergencies, or comply with government regulations and recommendations. Written reports are crucial to your Exposure Control Program and are, therefore, an important part of your daily routine.

Although you may not be directly responsible for maintaining the written reports required for your Exposure Control Program, your responsibility is to understand which reports are required, why they are necessary, and what your role is in keeping information up-to-date.

Exposure Control Program

Overall, the best report you can have is a sound, easily understood, and effectively implemented Exposure Control Program. The written portion of this program is centered around the Infection Control/Exposure Control Plan, which contains three types of written reports: procedures, records, and documentation.

	Report	Timing	Examples
1) Procedures	Written, step-by-step procedures accurately reflect tasks while integrating the many factors affecting your practice	Developed once, routinely reassessed, and changed when situations warrant	Standard Operating Procedures, Workplace Emergency Plans
2) Records	Records contain information useful in emergencies & help in determining who is at risk for Exposure Incidents	Information created for use in specific situations and updated as needed	Health Records, Chemical Inventory, Exposure Determination Charts, Training
3) Documentation	These are written reports, triggered by events and are used as support material or to fulfill, or verify, legal requirements	The form to document an event is developed in advance and forms are completed as a result of the event	Exposure Incidents, Waste Disposal, Biologic Monitoring, Evaluating Safer Sharps Devices

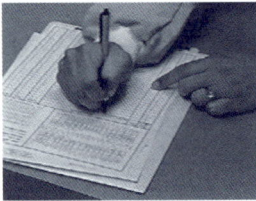

The written reports that a practice uses vary according to the location of the practice, number of employees, types of materials used, and types of procedures performed. They should also comply with any government regulations and recommendations from government agencies and professional organizations. Your practice uses written reports in the following areas:

Standard Operating Procedures:

These are step-by-step descriptions of how to perform daily tasks. Standard Operating Procedures (SOPs) have been discussed previously, primarily in Courses #4 and #5.

Employee Health Records:

These records are created at the time of initial employment and updated as indicated. They are referred to in emergency situations.

Employee Training Records:

These are used to document training. The form you sign at the end of each course and the test itself are examples.

Emergency Procedures Plans:

These procedures are developed prior to an emergency. You must be familiar with the plan and your role in an emergency. Included are the Postexposure Management Plans and the Workplace Emergency Procedures Plan, which are discussed in Course #2 and later in this course.

Chemical Safety Records:

The written requirements for chemical safety consist of all three types of reports: SOPs for tasks involving handling chemicals, records such as the Chemical Inventory and documentation for training, disposal, etc. Chemical safety is discussed in Course #8.

Dental Waste:

Your practice is responsible for all of the waste it generates. Manifests or disposal receipts are important means of proving your compliance with existing regulations. The handling, storage, and disposal of dental waste is covered in Course #9.

Miscellaneous:

Additional reports are necessary to document events that occur on a regular basis. These reports include: Sterilization Logs, Biologic Monitoring Logs, Dental Unit Waterline Maintenance Logs, Equipment Maintenance Logs, Housekeeping Logs and Evaluation of Safer Sharps.

Location of Written Reports

All employees should know the location of the Infection Control/Exposure Control Plan and all other related reports and documents. Your Infection Control/Exposure Control Plan should contain most of the required written reports, however, some may be in other locations. All written reports should be located where most efficient, and the location must be noted in the Infection Control/Exposure Control Plan.

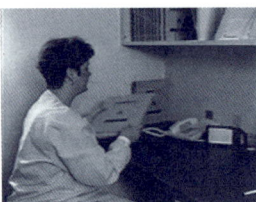

- **Reports may be maintained in a convenient location. A Biologic Monitoring Log located near the sterilizer is an example.**

- **Some reports are confidential and are kept in separate locked files, available only to employees with permission and some government agents. Examples include Employee Health Records and Exposure Incident Reports.**

- **Some information, due to the amount of data, such as the chemical Safety Data Sheets (SDS), may be kept in their own binder.**

This course will discuss written reports, what information they contain, where they may be kept, your role in using them, and how they may help you. You will need to locate some of these reports during the course. If you are unaware of the location of some reports, ask your Infection Control Coordinator or Safety Officer for assistance.

Note:

The reports you handle most often may be patient records. These are related to individual patients, customized by your practice, and impact your Exposure Control Plan when they are used to plan treatment for a specific procedure. We will not discuss patient records further in this section. If you have any questions concerning your practice's patient records, ask your Infection Control Coordinator or Safety Officer or other appropriate person.

Employee Health Records

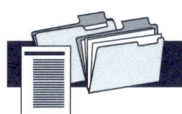

There are many different types of tasks that need to be performed in a dental practice, and subsequently, there are different levels of potential exposure risks for each employee. All employees share the same potential to be exposed to some hazards, such as fire or certain chemical vapors, however, the level of exposure to infectious or chemical hazards may vary. A bookkeeper or front desk employee who is never involved in clinical tasks, and never handles contaminated patient records, has a different potential for exposure than a clinical worker.

Infection Exposure Determination

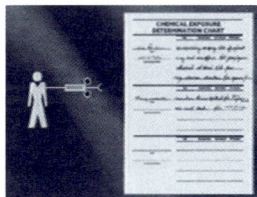

The Exposure Determination, covered in Course #2, is an identification of each individual employee who is at risk for on-the-job exposure to bloodborne pathogens. This information is documented in the Infection Control/Exposure Control Plan. If you have *any* contact with bloodborne pathogens, you are at risk for occupational exposure and are protected by the OSHA Bloodborne Pathogens Standard. Employees at-risk for infectious hazards are given training, offered the hepatitis B immunization series, and must have health records on file. It is important to know your potential exposure to infectious hazards.

Chemical Exposure Determination

Similar to the Exposure Determination, a Chemical Exposure Determination Chart may be used to determine your potential exposure to hazardous chemicals. If you have *any* contact with any hazardous chemical agents, you are covered by the OSHA Hazard Communications Standard and you have a right to know your risks, be trained in proper handling and emergency procedures, and be offered appropriate Personal Protective Equipment (PPE). A Chemical Exposure Determination Chart helps the Infection Control Coordinator or Safety Officer decide who is covered under the Hazard Communication Standard and which chemicals each employee uses. An employee working with hazardous chemicals is considered an at-risk employee and should fill out the appropriate health records. (Course #8)

Health records for employees at risk for on-the-job exposure to bloodborne pathogens are used by healthcare professionals to provide the optimal medical response in the event of any exposure incident. It is beneficial to keep your personal health record as complete as possible. These records should be filled out at the time of hire and reviewed at least annually, or if there is a change in your health status. They *may* contain the following information:

- **Your name, social security number and date of birth (required)**

- **Hepatitis B immunization status, or a waiver if you choose not to have the immunization (required)**

- **Status of other immunizations, such as measles, mumps, diphtheria, and tetanus as currently recommended by CDC Advisory Council on Immunization Practices (ACIP) The date of the last immunization should be noted for situations where a booster may be indicated. For example, the CDC now recommends that individuals vaccinated for Measles prior to 1957 should have their titer checked for evidence of immunity.**

**Acceptable evidence of immunity against measles includes at least one of the following: written documentation of adequate vaccination, laboratory evidence of immunity, laboratory confirmation of measles, or birth in the United States before 1957 www.cdc.gov/features/measles/index.html

- **TB status, Tuberculin Skin Testing (TST) screening results and follow-up as indicated**

- **Occupational exposure incident reports (if any)**

- **A physician's written follow-up report regarding the status of the hepatitis B immunization (optional)**

- **Allergies, or adverse reactions to any chemical agents or similar components**

- **Any drug allergies or contraindications to medical treatment**

- **Any other pertinent medical information that could impact follow-up treatment**

- **Whom to notify in an emergency, phone numbers and addresses**

If an exposure incident occurs, the following reports are added to the Employee Health Record to document the incident:

- **A report of the incident (if required):** The OSHA 301 Injury Report Form complies with the CDC injury reporting and documentation recommendations.Therefore, it may be advisable to use the OSHA 301 Form, even if your practice setting is exempted from the OSHA recordkeeping regulations. For more details on OSHA recordkeeping exemptions see information located toward the end of this course in the section titled "Work-Related Injury & Illness Record Keeping."

- **A list of any documents provided by your employer to the designated healthcare professional.**

- **The written opinion of the evaluating healthcare professional,** which identifies, within 15 days, whether a hepatitis B immunization was recommended for the exposed employee, whether or not the employee received the immunization, and whether that follow-up, if indicated, will occur.

Your health record is not to be used as an exposure incident report nor should it contain anything in addition to the written opinion of the evaluating Healthcare Professional, unless required by law.

Confidentiality of Records

After an exposure incident, the healthcare professional will inform you of the results of any tests and discuss your need for further medical treatment. The employee health record is a confidential document protected by federal and state-specific statutes and regulations. Test results and other recommendations for follow-up treatment are kept confidential and *are not placed* in your employee health record (unless you give informed consent to do so.

Location of Health Records

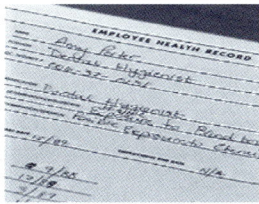

Employee health records are kept either on-site at the dental practice or with the designated healthcare professional throughout your term of employment and for a period of 30 years after your last day of employment. Generally, no one has access to any portion of your medical record besides yourself, your employer or someone designated by your employer (such as your Infection Control Coordinator or Safety Officer), and some government agencies. The release of any medical record, in any case, must comply with the appropriate state and federal laws that protect an individual's right to privacy.

Note:

If a portion of your medical record is kept at another location, such as a hospital or a healthcare professional's office, you or your legal representative may request permission to have access to your medical record. OSHA may request, as part of an investigation, a copy of your medical record.

Employees Not At-Risk

If you are not at-risk for exposure to infectious or chemical hazards, this information is documented during the Exposure Determination and no health record is necessary. However, it is prudent to have basic medical information on file for every employee in the event of an emergency. Periodically, your duties should be reviewed to ensure that they have not changed. If your duties have changed, you may need to update the Exposure Determination Charts and have a health record on file.

Training Documentation

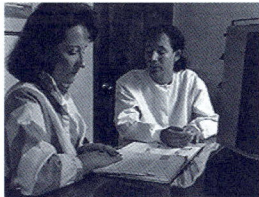

Training is fundamental to any efficient Exposure Control Program and the creation of a safe dental environment. A complete training program addresses the hazards you face in dentistry every day: infectious, physical, chemical, as well as hazards associated with waste management. Training must be documented to keep track of the employee's educational accomplishments as well as to verify compliance with required training. Maintain training records according to state and federal requirements.

Training Addresses All Hazards in Dentistry

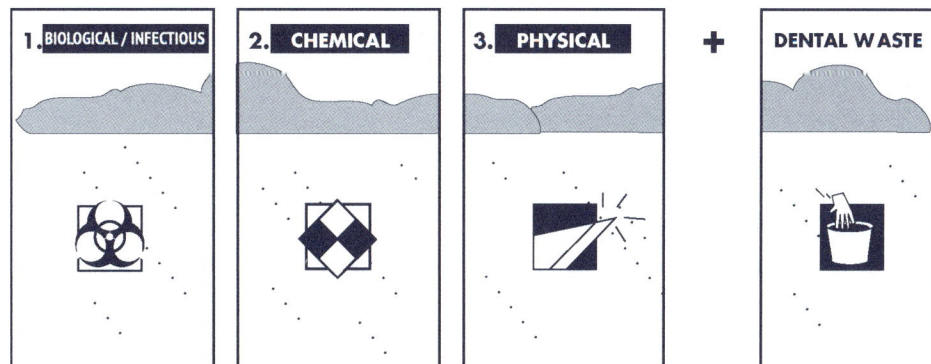

| 1. BIOLOGICAL / INFECTIOUS | 2. CHEMICAL | 3. PHYSICAL | + | DENTAL WASTE |

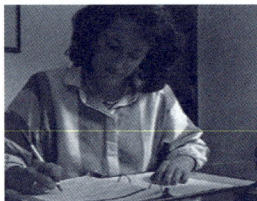

Documentation of training is completed after a training session or course is attended and must be kept for three years. These records should be placed in the Infection Control/Exposure Control Plan or filed by the Training Coordinator/ Infection Control Coordinator or Safety Officer. There should be blank forms available that are simply filled out at the end of each training session. Minimally they should include:

- **Date and length of the training session**
- **Who conducted the training and their qualifications** (your Infection Control Coordinator or Safety Officer or person facilitating training)
- **The names, job titles, and Social Security numbers or professional license numbers of all who attended**
- **Content of training**

Some dental practices may ask that you sign a form verifying that you did indeed attend and complete a particular training program. A copy of this form will be kept with the training documentation. In addition, a copy of an off-site course/ seminar confirmation form may be required.

Note:

Occasionally, to ensure compliance with OSHA training standards, a representative from OSHA may request copies of training records.

Chemical Safety Records

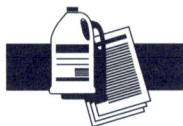

The chemicals you use in a dental practice may pose serious health risks. Under the OSHA Hazard Communications Standard, chemical agents that are determined to be hazardous or potentially hazardous to employees must be handled and disposed according to industry guidelines and/or methods established by manufacturers.

Chemical Inventory

The most basic chemical safety record is a list of all the chemicals used in your practice. This Chemical Inventory should be updated on a regular basis and each year's inventory must be kept for 30 years. A complete Chemical Inventory is essential for an effective chemical safety program.

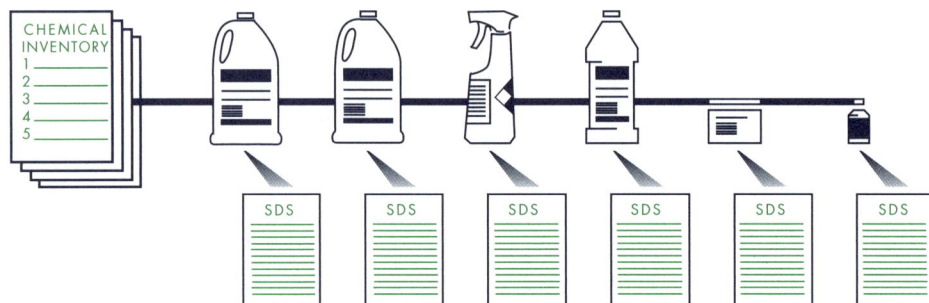

Each chemical on the inventory must have a corresponding Safety Data Sheet (SDS) on file. SDSs are documents that describe the ingredients, hazards, and emergency procedures for each chemical. Manufacturers and importers are required to prepare an SDS for each hazardous product they produce or import, and distributors must relay this information to the users. You must know the location of the SDS file, and how to read and interpret the information it provides.

Given the variety of chemicals in any practice, it is critical to document their use and disposal, especially since all chemicals are not disposed of in the same manner (Course #9). Examples include:

- **Immersion Chemical Sterilant Log**
- **Hazardous Waste Disposal Manifest (e.g., spent fixer, expired hazardous chemicals, etc.)**

These records are used to prove compliance and to verify, for the practice, when and how events took place.

Chemical Exposure Determination

The Hazard Communication Standard training requirements differ from the Bloodborne Pathogens Standard, since training is specific to the chemical agent and the individual handling or expected to handle that agent. A Chemical Exposure Determination Chart helps evaluate your potential chemical exposure based on which chemical agents you use or are in contact with during the day and determines your training needs.

All employees must have some general knowledge of chemical handling, safety, and emergency response in the event of an exposure or spill. However, more intense training may be required depending on the chemical. For example, while all clinical workers may need to be trained on the proper use, mixing, and storage of disinfectants used in operatory processing, only employees who process radiographic films are required to be specifically trained for the use of radiographic processing chemicals.

Workplace Emergency Procedures

Do you know what to do in the event of an emergency in the office? Where is the nearest exit or fire extinguisher? Where is the eyewash station? What happens if a patient slips and is injured? What should you do in the event of a chemical or blood spill?

Plan: Written Or Oral

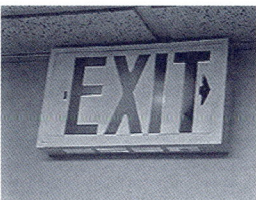

Workplace emergencies are covered in a Comprehensive Emergency Procedure Plan. For most states, a written plan is required for companies with 11 or more employees. If your practice has 10 or fewer employees, you still need a plan, but it can be communicated orally to employees. Your role in an emergency may be crucial to the safety of yourself or others. To be effective, a workplace emergency plan requires the support of all employees. You should be familiar enough with your practice's plan to answer the following questions:

How many exits are there for your facility? _____   *Are they labeled?* _____ **(There should be at least two clearly labeled exits)**

7 · 8

In the event of an emergency evacuation, is there equipment that must be shut down, and, if so, who is assigned to accomplish this?

Equipment: _____

Responsibility: _____

Equipment: _____

Responsibility: _____

Equipment: _____

Responsibility: _____

What is the procedure for evacuating patients:

Under Sedation? _____

With a Treatment Wound? _____

With a Rubber Dam? _____

Where do you meet to account for everyone after evacuation?

_____

How do you report a fire or other emergency?

_____

Where are your fire blanket and fire extinguisher(s)?

_____

What are your responsibilities during a fire or other emergency?

_____

Where are the first aid kit(s) and medical emergency equipment?

_____

Where are the accident report forms?

_____

Whom do you contact for information concerning your practice's fire and emergency plan?

_____

Physical Emergencies

The Comprehensive Emergency Procedure Plan should address all potential emergencies, including:

- Emergency escape procedures and exit routes
- Procedures for critical operations that must be performed before evacuation
- Procedures to account for all employees and patients after an emergency evacuation
- Rescue and medical duties
- Means of reporting fires and other emergencies
- Contacts for information or clarification

Your employer and/or Infection Control Coordinator or Safety Officer should routinely perform a hazard audit to identify unsafe and potentially unsafe conditions. You, and other employees, should always report unsafe conditions. Many of these conditions can be addressed as a way to *prevent* workplace emergencies. Some examples include:

Housekeeping:
The place of employment must be kept clean and uncluttered.

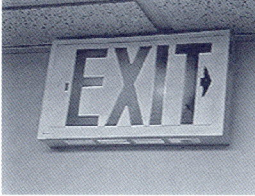

Exits:
There must be at least two clearly marked, unlocked exits, kept free of all obstructions. If an exit needs artificial light, then light must be provided.

Electrical Equipment:
Electrical equipment needs to be grounded. If any wiring is faulty, worn, or otherwise compromised, it needs to be replaced. Extension cords used for permanent fixtures should be replaced with fixed wiring.

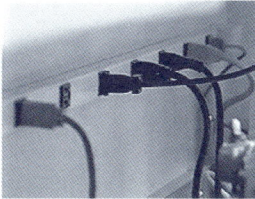

Compressed Gas Cylinders:
These should be properly secured (using chain or wire), not stored near solid materials that burn rapidly or near exits, stairways, or in areas normally used, or intended to be used, for the safe exit of people. The area should have minimal exposure to excessive temperatures, physical damage, or tampering. Containers should be labeled to reflect usage and empty containers should be stored outside. If stored inside, they must be considered full.

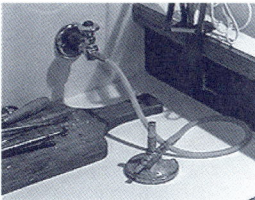

Ventilation:
A local exhaust ventilation system must be present and maintained, whenever dry grinding, dry polishing, or buffing is performed, and if the exposure (without the use of respirators) exceeds the permissible exposure limits. Ventilation may also be required for chemicals such as glutaraldehydes or formaldehydes.

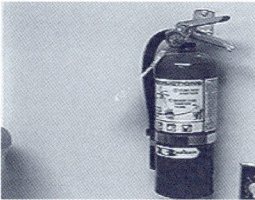

Flammable Vapors:
Precautions must be taken when working with flammable vapors; they must not be used around open flames or other sources of ignition.

Fire Extinguishers:
Fire extinguishers must be visually inspected each month, placed a maximum of 75 feet from any location, and employees should be trained in their proper use. If an automatic sprinkler system is installed, it must be properly maintained.

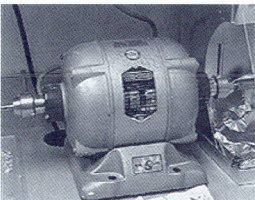

Air Compressor Drains and Traps:
The drain valve on the air receiver shall be opened and the receiver completely drained frequently and at such intervals as to prevent the accumulation of excessive amounts of liquid in the receiver.

Dental Lathes:
Machines designed to be anchored must be securely fixed. Safety shields must be used to prevent physical injuries.

These items and any potentially unsafe conditions should be reviewed and any problems corrected. The manner in which the review is conducted is part of the written plan.

Medical emergencies deserve special note. Although injuries or sudden illnesses of patients or employees may be rare in dentistry, your employer should ensure that one person on each shift is trained in first aid and cardiopulmonary resuscitation (CPR). First aid equipment must be kept at the office with its contents updated periodically, and checked for proper working order and for expiration dates. To provide appropriate and immediate medical care, arrangements should be made with a local emergency healthcare facility, *prior* to any emergency. This should be part of your emergency plan.

Chemical Emergencies

Chemical spills can cause two problems: potential fire and/or explosion, and potential health hazards. The SDSs contain information about the flammability or combustibility associated with each chemical used in the practice, as well as any health hazards. All staff should be familiar with procedures for reporting and cleaning up a spill and the first aid procedures indicated for that chemical. These directions are provided on the SDS and must be followed carefully.

Work-Related Injury & Illness Record Keeping

OSHA Forms 300 and 301

Many, but not all employers are required to complete the OSHA injury and illness recordkeeping forms 300 (log of work-related injuries and illness) and 301 (summary of work-related injuries and illness). Exceptions as of January 1, 2015, include:

- Small employer exemption – 10 or fewer employees at all times during the year

- Low-hazard industry exemption (Partially Exempt Industries) - dental offices are included in the list of Partially Exempt Industries (NAICS #6212 Offices of Dentist)

Certain incidents must be reported to OSHA, even if a business has fewer than 10 employees or is categorized as a low-hazard industry. This includes dental offices. All employers, including those partially exempted by reason of company size or industry classification, must report to OSHA any workplace incident that results in a fatality, in-patient hospitalization, amputation, or loss of an eye. For more information, visit the OSHA injury and illness recordkeeping and reporting requirements web page: www.osha.gov/recordkeeping/index.html

Please note that if a dental office is part of a hospital or larger health institution, it may need to keep records using the OSHA forms. States with OSHA-approved plans may require employers to keep records such as OSHA form 300 (log of work-related injuries and illness) and 301 (summary of work-related injuries and illness) even if the federal OSHA program exempts them. There are also states which may have specific recordkeeping requirements for injuries associated with contaminated sharps. This varies from state to state and is regulated through a variety of state agencies including departments of public health. It is important to check your state regulations as well as any pertinent Board of Registration in Dentistry requirements

For more information on OSHA recordkeeping requirements, visit these OSHA weblinks:
OSHA Illness and Injury Recordkeeping resource page:
www.osha.gov/recordkeeping/index.html

Certain low-risk industries are exempted:
www.osha.gov/recordkeeping/ppt1/RK1exempttable.html

State -specific recordkeeping requirements for State-specific OSHA plans:
www.osha.gov/dcsp/osp/index.html

Regulations (Standards - 29 CFR) General recording criteria. - 1904.7

1904.7(a) *Basic requirement.* You must consider an injury or illness to meet the general recording criteria, and therefore to be recordable, if it results in any of the following: death, days away from work, restricted work or transfer to another job, medical treatment beyond first aid, or loss of consciousness. You must also consider a case to meet the general recording criteria if it involves a significant injury or illness diagnosed by a physician or other licensed healthcare professional, even if it does not result in death, days away from work, restricted work or job transfer, medical treatment beyond first aid, or loss of consciousness. (www.osha.gov/pls/oshaweb/owadisp.show_document?p_table=STANDARDS&p_id=9638)

OSHA Poster 3165

This poster outlines the rights of an employee in any given situation and must be posted at all times in an employee area. www.osha.gov/Publications/poster.html

CDC Recommendations for Documentation and Recordkeeping of Work-Related Injury and Illnesses

The health status of DHCP can be monitored by maintaining records of work-related medical evaluations, screening tests, immunizations, exposures, and postexposure management. Such records must be kept in accordance with all applicable state and federal laws. Examples of laws that might apply include the Privacy Rule of the Health Insurance Portability and Accountability Act (HIPAA) of 1996, 45 CFR 160 and 164, and the OSHA Occupational Exposure to Blood-borne Pathogens; Final Rule 29 CFR 1910.1030(h)(1)(i--iv) (34,13). The HIPAA Privacy Rule applies to covered entities, including certain defined health providers, healthcare clearinghouses, and health plans.

CDC recommendations include the development of policies and procedures for prompt reporting, evaluation, counseling, treatment and medical follow-up of occupational exposures. Dental settings should be prepared to respond to work-related injuries and illness and provide care as soon as possible. After an occupational blood exposure, first aid should be administered as necessary. Exposed DHCP should immediately report the exposure to the Infection Control Coordinator or other designated person, who should initiate referral to the qualified healthcare professional and complete necessary reports. Because multiple factors contribute to the risk of infection after an occupational exposure to blood, the following information should be included in the exposure report, recorded in the exposed person's confidential medical record, and provided to the qualified healthcare professional:

- **Date and time of exposure.**
- **Details of the procedure being performed, including where and how the exposure occurred and whether the exposure involved a sharp device, the type and brand of device, and how and when during its handling the exposure occurred.**
- **Details of the exposure, including its severity and the type and amount of fluid or material. For a percutaneous injury, severity might be measured by the depth of the wound, gauge of the needle, and whether fluid was injected; for a skin or mucous membrane exposure, the estimated volume of material, duration of contact, and the condition of the skin (e.g., chapped, abraded, or intact) should be noted.**
- **Details regarding whether the source material was known to contain HIV or other bloodborne pathogens, and, if the source was infected with HIV, the stage of disease, history of antiretroviral therapy, and viral load, if known.**
- **Details regarding the exposed person (e.g., hepatitis B vaccination and vaccine-response status).**
- **Details regarding counseling, postexposure management, and follow-up.**
- **The susceptibility of the exposed person.**

In addition to exposure records, thorough recordkeeping of all work-related injuries and illness can be especially helpful if an illness or injury later results in complications or is determined to be an infectious disease exposure. OSHA forms 300 (log of work-related injuries and illness) and 301 (summary of work-related injuries and illness) can be used to record and describe injuries and illnesses. OSHA has specific illness and injury recordkeeping rules for employers that require use of these forms.

Note:

OSHA requires employers to ensure that certain information contained in employee medical records is 1) kept confidential; 2) not disclosed or reported without the employee's express written consent to any person within or outside the workplace except as required by the OSHA standard; and 3) maintained by the employer for at least the duration of employment plus 30 years. Dental practices that coordinate their infection-control program with off-site providers might consult OSHA's Bloodborne Pathogen standard and employee Access to Medical and Exposure Records standard, as well as other applicable local, state, and federal laws, to determine a location for storing health records.

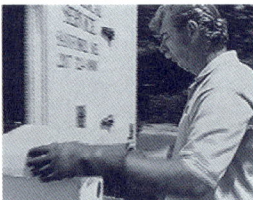

Dental Waste Record Keeping

All dental offices generate hazardous and general waste. Hazardous waste can be an infectious, chemical, or physical (sharps) hazard or any combination of these. What records you keep is determined by the type of waste generated and your method of disposal. Your practice is responsible for much of the dental waste it generates from "cradle to grave," or until the waste is ultimately destroyed and/or rendered nonhazardous.

Record keeping for waste generally follows two paths: chemical waste and infectious waste. A Dental Waste Management Plan details the steps to ensure that the infectious and chemical waste generated in your practice is appropriately handled and disposed in accordance with federal, state and local requirements. Since your office is ultimately responsible for the proper disposal of hazardous waste, careful records must be kept regarding its disposal.

This record is a manifest (tracking document and detailed receipt) and may contain:
- **A description of the waste**
- **Total quantity of waste being shipped**
- **The type of container used in shipping**
- **Transporter name and address**
- **Transporter state permit or ID number**
- **Quantity and category of waste transported**
- **Date of shipment**
- **A signature of the representative accepting the waste for shipment**

The manifest is provided by the hazardous waste disposal company. Records, policies, and documentation are required for on-site treatment of infectious waste. These include an SOP for waste sterilization, Biologic Monitoring Logs for each infectious waste sterilization load, and equipment maintenance records. Dental waste disposal will be covered in Course #9.

Monitoring, Maintenance and Housekeeping Records

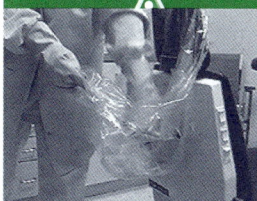

Additional reports are useful for housekeeping. There are various tasks, performed on a routine basis, where it is desirable to document the event to prove compliance, to maintain quality and to troubleshoot if a problem is detected. These reports include:

1. Sterilization Monitoring Log:
Documents the date, load number, and if more than one sterilizer, which sterilizer was used. If there is ever a problem associated with sterilization, this log helps to identify potentially improperly sterilized packages so they can be repackaged and resterilized.

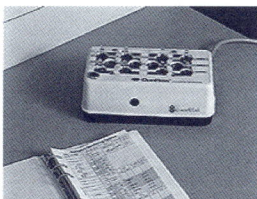

2. Biologic Monitoring Log:
Routine biologic monitoring of each sterilizer is a critical component of any sterility assurance program. This log records all relevant data for each biologic monitoring step. Many mail-in monitoring services as well as in-office biologic monitoring equipment companies provide these logs to their customers. The log should minimally have the following:
- Date
- Load number
- Parameters for sterilization (temperature, pressure, time, etc.)
- Who placed the Biological Indicator (BI) in the sterilizer
- The Control BI and Test BI result

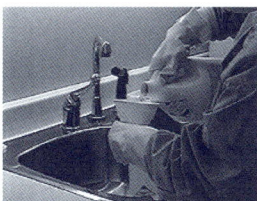

3. Equipment Maintenance and Repair:
A list of dates for equipment maintenance and repair. Receipts and service contracts should also be filed.

4. Dental Unit Water Quality Maintenance Log:
Follow the manufacturer's instructions for the specific dental unit water quality product/device manufacturer's instructions.

5. Housekeeping Schedule:
A form to fill out to verify that the office environment and equipment are appropriately cleaned and maintained on a regular basis.

Evaluation of Safer Sharps Documentation

The evaluation of sharps with engineered safety features, covered in Course #2, addresses the November 6, 2000, Needlestick Safety Prevention Act that caused the revision of 1991 Bloodborne Standards in 2001. In addition to the other provisions of the 1991 standard, employers are required by OSHA to document (1) annual consideration and implementation of appropriate engineering controls [definition of engineering controls updated and includes, but is not limited to, "safer medical devices, such as sharps with engineered sharps injury protections and needleless systems."], and (2) solicitation of employee input in evaluating and choosing devices.

To do this, dentist-employers must:
- **stay abreast of innovations in procedures and technological developments that reduce the risk of occupational exposures (i.e., newly available devices designed to reduce sharps injuries); and**
- **document consideration and/or of appropriate, commercially available and effective safer devices, for example, by describing the devices identified as candidates for use, the method(s) used to assess their feasibility, and justification for the decision to use or not use the devices.**

To demonstrate compliance with the revised standard, employers must document solicitation of input from employees in the written Exposure Control Program. OSHA suggests two possible ways of documenting compliance:
- **listing the employees involved and describing the process by which input was requested, or**
- **through other documentation, such as references to meeting minutes, copies of documents used to request employee participation, or records of responses received from employees.**

Course #2 outlines a method for identifying, screening and evaluating safer devices and provides links to CDC sample forms.

Sense of Security

The reports used in your practice help monitor your practice's exposure control program. Incomplete reports do not necessarily mean unsafe conditions. Complete and accurate recordkeeping will help ensure the safest dental visit for you and your patients.

Examples of Major Documentation

Required - OSHA

1. Written Plans:
- Bloodborne Pathogens
- Hazard Communication
- Emergency Procedures
- Waste Management

2. **Employee Health Records**

3. **Employee Training Records**

4. **Incident Reports:** (if any) Form 301/300 or state equivalents, Workers Compensation forms, etc.

5. **Exposure Determination Charts:** Bloodborne Pathogens, Chemical, Other

6. **Safer Sharps Evaluation Documentation**

7. **SDSs, Chemical Inventory**

8. **Other**

Required — EPA/State/Local Waste Regulations

1. **Waste disposal records**

2. **Waste disposal manifests**

3. **Other**

Other Important Documentation (unless otherwise specified by state law)

1. **Worksheet on Hazard Abatement**

2. **Housekeeping Schedule**

3. **Environmental Surface Disinfection Log**

4. **High-level Disinfection Log**

5. **Biologic Monitoring Logs**

6. **Equipment Maintenance Schedule**

7. **Records/receipts for equipment repairs**

8. **Schedule of implementation dates for time-specific activities.** Examples include biologic monitoring, cleaning and changing chemicals in developer, and instrument inventory.

Other Practice-Specific Records (Fill in the Blanks for Any Additional Records Your Practice May Use)

1. _____

2. _____

3. _____

4. _____

5. _____

⚠ Discussion

Discuss with your Infection Control Coordinator or Safety Officer your responsibilities for documentation and recordkeeping including what checklists should be used.

Objectives

Upon completion of this course on hazard communication, you will be able to:

1. Describe the procedure for responding to a chemical incident.

2. Describe the three steps of a Hazard Communications Program.

3. Identify the five components of a chemical Hazard Communication Program.

4. Identify the meaning of each pictogram used with the hazard communication warning system.

5. Define and understand each section of the SDS (Safety Data Sheet).

6. List three labeling requirements of a chemical product.

7. Demonstrate proper management of a chemical exposure to the eyes.

Focus

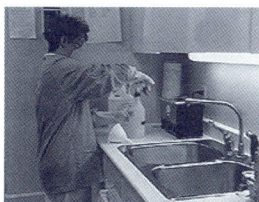

DHCP are exposed to potentially hazardous chemicals. From glutaraldehyde, to nitrous oxide, to chlorine bleach, to common sink cleaners, the list encompasses a large variety of chemicals. Each chemical has its own procedures for safe preparation, use, clean up, disposal, and emergency response.

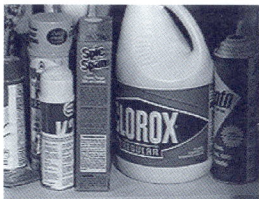

The Hazard Communication Standard (HCS) was adopted by OSHA in 1989 to address hazards associated with chemicals in the workplace. Referred to as the "Right-to-Know Law," or "HAZCOM," this standard is based on a simple concept – as an employee, you have both a need and a right to know the identities of the chemicals "known to be present" while working, as well as their hazards and what protective measures are available, and should be provided to you, to prevent adverse effects from occurring.

Hazard Communication Standard Gets Revised

In 2012, OSHA modified the Hazard Communication Standard to align with the Globally Harmonized System of Classification and Labeling of Chemicals (GHS). The GHS provides an internationally accepted, standardized format for chemical classification, product labels and safety data sheets. The parts of the 1989 HCS that did not relate to the GHS such as the basic framework, scope, and exemptions remained largely unchanged. There have been some modifications to terminology in order to align with the GHS. For example, the term "hazard determination" has been changed to "hazard classification" and "material safety data sheet" (MSDS) was changed to "safety data sheet" (SDS).

Following is a brief overview of the major changes in the revised Hazard Communication Standard (HCS):

1. **Hazard Classification** - provides specific criteria for classification of health and physical hazards, as well as classification of mixtures;

2. **Labels** - chemical manufacturers and importers are required to provide a label that includes a harmonized signal word, pictogram and hazard statement for each hazard class and category, and precautionary statements must also be provided; (see HCS Pictograms and Hazards on pages that follow);

3. **Safety Data Sheets (SDS)** - formerly known as Material Safety Data Sheets, have a specified 16-section format (see SDS format requirements on pages that follow);

4. **Information and training** - employers are required to train employees on the new label elements and safety data sheets format to facilitate recognition and understanding.

For a side-by-side comparison of the current HCS and the final revised HCS please see OSHA's hazard communication safety and health topics webpage at: www.osha.gov/dsg/hazcom/side-by-side.html

Effective Dates For Implementation of the Updated Standard

1. Employers shall train employees regarding the new label elements and safety data sheets format by December 1, 2013. See OSHA Fact Sheet "December 1, 2013 Training Requirements for the Revised Hazard Communication Standard" at: www.osha.gov/Publications/OSHA3642.pdf

2. Chemical manufacturers, importers, distributors, and employers shall be in compliance with all modified provisions of this section no later than June 1, 2015, except:

   • After December 1, 2015, the distributor shall not ship containers labeled by the chemical manufacturer or importer unless the label has been modified to comply with the standard.

   • All employers shall, as necessary, update any alternative workplace labeling, update the hazard communication program, and provide any additional employee training for newly identified physical or health hazards no later than June 1, 2016.

3. Chemical manufacturers, importers, distributors, and employers may comply with either the old or the current version of this standard, or both during the transition period.

Effective Completion Date	Requirement(s)	Who
December 1, 2013	Train employees on the new label elements and safety data sheet (SDS) format.	Employers
June 1, 2015	Compliance with all modified provisions of this final rule, except:	Chemical manufacturers, importers, distributors and employers
December 1, 2015	The Distributor shall not ship containers labeled by the chemical manufacturer or importer unless it is a GHS label.	
June 1, 2016	Update alternative workplace labeling and hazard communication program as necessary, and provide additional employee training for newly identified physical or health hazards.	Employers
Transition Period to the effective completion dates noted above	May comply with either 29 CFR 1910.1200 (the final standard), or the current standard, or both.	Chemical manufacturers, importers, distributors, and employers

Revised Standard for Classification and Labels – HCS Pictogram

As of June 1, 2015, the Hazard Communication Standard (HCS) requires pictograms on labels to alert users of the chemical hazards to which they may be exposed. Each pictogram consists of a symbol on a white background framed within a red border and represents a distinct hazard(s). The pictogram on the label is determined by the chemical hazard classification. The standard specifies what information is to be provided for each hazard class and category. Labels will require the following elements:

- **Pictogram:** a symbol plus other graphic elements, such as a border, background pattern, or color that is intended to convey specific information about the hazards of a chemical. Each pictogram consists of a different symbol on a white background within a red square frame set on a point (i.e. a red diamond). There are nine pictograms under the GHS. However, only eight pictograms are required under the HCS, the exception being the environmental pictogram, as environmental hazards are not within OSHA's jurisdiction.

- **Signal words**: a single word used to indicate the relative level of severity of hazard and alert the reader to a potential hazard on the label. The signal words used are "danger" and "warning." "Danger" is used for the more severe hazards, while "warning" is used for less severe hazards.

- **Hazard Statement:** a statement assigned to a hazard class and category that describes the nature of the hazard(s) of a chemical, including, where appropriate, the degree of hazard.

- **Precautionary Statement:** a phrase that describes recommended measures to be taken to minimize or prevent adverse effects resulting from exposure to a hazardous chemical, or improper storage or handling of a hazardous chemical.

HCS Pictograms and Hazards

Health Hazard

- Carcinogen
- Mutagenicity
- Reproductive Toxicity
- Respiratory Sensitizer
- Target Organ Toxicity
- Aspiration Toxicity

Flame

- Flammables
- Pyrophorics
- Self-Heating
- Emits Flammable Gas
- Self-Reactives
- Organic Peroxides

Exclamation Mark

- Irritant (skin and eye)
- Skin Sensitizer
- Acute Toxicity (harmful)
- Narcotic Effects
- Respiratory Tract Irritant
- Hazardous to Ozone Layer (Non-Mandatory)

Gas Cylinder

- Gases Under Pressure

Corrosion

- Skin Corrosion/Burns
- Eye Damage
- Corrosive to Metals

Exploding Bomb

- Explosives
- Self-Reactives
- Organic Peroxides

Flame Over Circle

- Oxidizers

Environment (Non-Mandatory)

- Aquatic Toxicity

Skull and Crossbones

- Acute Toxicity (fatal or toxic)

Note: The pictogram above is posted so that you have a better understanding of the new labeling system. It is not accurate in that the representative chemical hazard symbol should be surrounded by a <u>RED diamond border.</u> A version of HCS pictograms and hazards with the red border can be found at this link: www.osha.gov/Publications/HazComm_QuickCard_Pictogram.html

Revised Standard and Workplace Relabeling

The current standard provides employers with flexibility regarding the type of system to be used in their workplaces and OSHA has retained that flexibility in the revised Hazard Communication Standard (HCS). Employers may choose to label workplace containers either with the same label that would be on shipped containers for the chemical under the revised rule, or with label alternatives that meet the requirements for the standard. Alternative labeling systems such as the National Fire Protection Association (NFPA) 704 Hazard Rating and the Hazardous Material Information System (HMIS) are permitted for workplace containers. However, the information supplied on these labels must be consistent with the revised HCS, e.g., no conflicting hazard warnings or pictograms.

OSHA® QUICK CARD™

Hazard Communication Standard Labels

OSHA has updated the requirements for labeling of hazardous chemicals under its Hazard Communication Standard (HCS). All labels are required to have pictograms, a signal word, hazard and precautionary statements, the product identifier, and supplier identification. A sample revised HCS label, identifying the required label elements, is shown on the right. Supplemental information can also be provided on the label as needed.

For more information:

OSHA® Occupational Safety and Health Administration
U.S. Department of Labor   www.osha.gov   (800) 321-OSHA (6742)

OSHA 3492-01R 2016

Revised Standard and Safety Data Sheet (SDS)

The information required on the safety data sheet (SDS) will remain essentially the same as that in the current standard. The current standard indicates what information has to be included on an SDS, but does not specify a format for presentation or order of information. The revised Hazard Communication Standard (HazCom 2012) requires that the information on the SDS be presented using specific headings in a specified sequence. The SDS format is the same as the ANSI standard format, which is widely used in the U.S. and is already familiar to many employees.

Safety Data Sheet (SDS) means written or printed material concerning a hazardous chemical that contains the following information:

1. **Identification** – includes product identifier; manufacturer or distributor name, address, phone number; emergency phone number; recommended use; restrictions on use.

2. **Hazard(s) identification** – includes all hazards regarding the chemical; required label elements.

3. **Composition/information on ingredients** – includes information on chemical ingredients; trade secret claims.

4. **First-aid measures** – includes important symptoms/effects, acute, delayed; required treatment.

5. **Fire-fighting measures** – lists suitable extinguishing techniques, equipment; chemical hazards from fire.

6. **Accidental release measures** – lists emergency procedures, protective equipment; proper methods of containment and cleanup.

7. **Handling and storage** – lists precautions for safe handling and storage, including incompatibilities.

8. **Exposure controls/personal protection** – lists OSHA's Permissible Exposure Limits (PELs); Threshold Limit Values (TLVs); appropriate engineering controls; personal protective equipment (PPE).

9. **Physical and chemical properties** – lists the chemical's characteristics.

10. **Stability and reactivity** – lists chemical stability and possibility of hazardous reactions.

11. **Toxicological information** – includes routes of exposure; related symptoms, acute and chronic effects; numerical measures of toxicity.

12. **Ecological information***

13. **Disposal considerations***

14. **Transport information***

15. **Regulatory information***

16. **Other information** – includes the date of preparation or last revision.

*Since other Agencies regulate this information, OSHA will not be enforcing Sections 12 through 15(29 CFR 1910.1200(g)(2).

OSHA believes that use of a consistent format will improve the effectiveness of SDSs by making information easier for the reader to find, regardless of the supplier of the SDS. Because the 16-section format is accepted by consensus as the most appropriate format, OSHA no longer endorses that Form 174 be used for the preparation of SDSs. Use of Form 174, however, is still acceptable under the HCS if it is completed correctly.

See Appendix D of 1910.1200 for a detailed description of SDS contents. (www.osha.gov/dsg/hazcom/hazcom-appendix-d.html). OSHA is preparing a guidance document that will include instructions for composing individual sections of the SDS. The guidance document will be posted on the OSHA website in the near future.

Notes to Employers

- The Hazard Communication Standard indicates that employers shall have a Safety Data Sheet in the workplace for each hazardous chemical used. (OSHA)[1]

- Employers must ensure that SDSs are readily accessible to employees. (OSHA)[1]

- The Bloodborne Pathogens Standard indicates that the written Exposure Control Plan shall be reviewed and updated at least annually and whenever necessary to reflect new or modified tasks or procedures. (OSHA)[2] This kind of review should also be applied to your Chemical Hazard Communication Program.

Links to Resources:

[1] OSHA. 29CFR Part 1910.2000, Hazard Communication Standard. Accessed May 2019 at: www.osha.gov/dsg/hazcom/HCSFinalRegTxt.html

[2] OSHA. CFR29 1910.1030, Bloodborne Pathogens Standard. Accessed May 2019 at: www.osha.gov/laws-regs/regulations/standardnumber/1910/1910.1030

Chemical Hazard Communications Program

A Chemical Hazard Communication Program has five main parts:

1. Written Program:
Describes who is covered as well as how to handle hazardous chemicals, comply with government regulations, and respond to emergencies.

2. Chemical Inventory:
A list of all of the chemicals in use.

3. Safety Data Sheets (SDS):
One SDS is required for each chemical agent in the inventory. These contain details you may need when working with hazardous chemicals.

4. Container Labeling:
Containers must be labeled to indicate, at the point of use, what they contain and any hazards that may be present.

5. Employee Training:
Employees must be trained specifically for the chemicals they will use, *prior* to use and *as necessary* to ensure safe use. To facilitate recognition and understanding, employees are also required to be trained by December 1, 2013, on the new label elements and Safety Data Sheet (SDS) format introduced in the 2012 update of he Hazard Communication Standard.

The development and maintenance of a Hazard Communication Program involves three steps – hazard assessment, hazard abatement, and hazard containment. In other words, first find out what the hazards are, then plan how to minimize the hazards and, finally, plan what to do in emergency situations to minimize additional harm. www.osha.gov/dsg/hazcom/index.html

Three Steps for the Hazard Communication Program

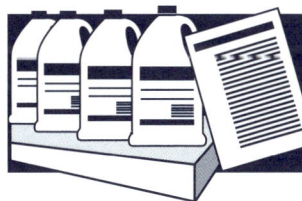

Hazard Assessment   **Hazard Abatement**   **Hazard Containment**

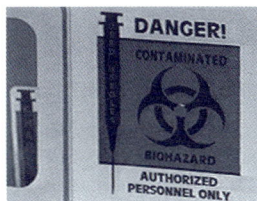

1 · Hazard Assessment involves listing all of the chemicals used in the practice and identifying the ingredients, hazards, and emergency procedures associated with each one. This process is accomplished by developing a Chemical Inventory and obtaining the corresponding and up-to-date SDS www.osha.gov/laws-regs/regulations/standardnumber/1910/1910.1030.

2 · Hazard Abatement involves the communication and understanding of hazards through employee training, container labels, and signs. Establishing appropriate Engineering and Work Practice Controls and providing appropriate PPE for the specific chemicals in use, are also means of hazard abatement.

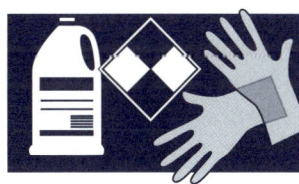

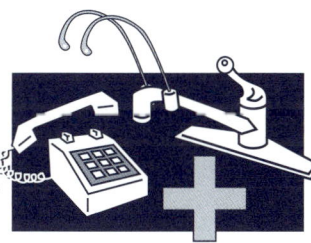

3 · Hazard Containment involves establishing emergency procedures for exposure incidents. Your Postexposure Management Plan contains a Chemical Exposure Incident Plan for hazard containment and follow-up.

Chemical Specific

The Hazard Communication Standard considers all chemicals as potentially dangerous but is *chemical-specific* on precautions. Each chemical used must have a corresponding SDS that outlines the specific hazards, safe limits of exposure, safe handling, disposal methods, and emergency procedures associated with that chemical. Training is also chemical-specific, as it informs you what PPE and Engineering and Work Practice Controls are necessary for safe use of each specific chemical you may use.

Locate your practice's written Hazard Communication Program in your practice's Infection Control/Exposure Control Plan.

Take the time to read it and understand what roles and responsibilities you and others have to ensure the safe use of chemicals.

Hazard Assessment

The first step in managing hazardous chemicals is to develop and implement a written, comprehensive Hazard Communication Program. This program should include provisions for identifying hazardous chemicals, determining who is at risk, collecting SDSs, labeling containers, and training employees. It should identify who is responsible for maintaining each portion of the plan, timetables for updating the information, and the location of the Chemical Inventory and SDSs.

Chemical Inventory

The next step is to identify the chemicals in use and develop the Chemical Inventory. This list should be accessible to all employees and must include the name of the hazardous chemical and a reference number for each chemical. This reference number then should be placed on the SDS to assist employees in quickly locating the appropriate SDS in an emergency. Other information included in the inventory may vary; however, the following may be useful:

- **Trade Name**
- **Chemical Name**
- **Where and how the chemical is used**
- **Date added to practice (or added to list) and date discontinued if appropriate (save all old lists and corresponding SDSs as a record in your files)**

Where is the Chemical Inventory kept in your practice?

The Chemical Inventory must be reviewed at least annually and updated when any new chemicals are introduced or removed from the work site. Updates must also occur when the brand of a chemical is changed. Depending on state and local regulations, this list may have to be provided annually to your local or state Department of Environmental Protection or Environmental Protection Agency.

Exposures to a chemical agent may have an immediate, delayed, or long-term health effect. All chemical records should be kept as a reference for future use. OSHA requires that each year's chemical records (SDS, Chemical Inventory, etc.) must be kept for a period of 30 years. If a practice is terminated, rather than sold to another individual, these records are then transferred to the director of the National Institute of Occupational Safety and Health (NIOSH).

Tips & Hints

- **Software programs are available to help you maintain your SDS and Chemical Inventory. A hard copy should be accessible in the event of the loss of power.**

- **The hard copy of your chemical records needs to be organized in a manner so that all staff can access them at any time. For example, the SDS may be alphabetically ordered by product name. You may also want to have a coding system to cross-reference like chemicals. For example, if iodine is a major ingredient in several products, you may want to cross-reference these products.**

- **The Chemical Inventory also indicates the primary use of the product, such as surface disinfectant, developer, etc.**

Exemptions

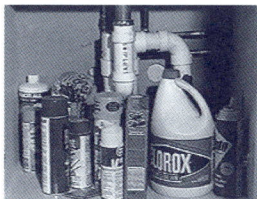

The Consumer Products Exemption Category allows some household products to be excluded from the Hazard Communication Standard. However, if household chemicals, such as chlorine bleach or scouring powder, are used in excess of household use or in a different form, concentration, or manner than generally used by consumers, they must be included on this list. For example, if you use a scouring powder all day long to clean sinks, you are exposed to it more frequently than if you used the product at home. The scouring powder would then need to have an SDS on file, be appropriately labeled, and employees trained on proper use of the product. Routine use of household products for professional use is not an acceptable alternative to implementing and managing a Hazard Communication Program.

Chemical Exposure Determination

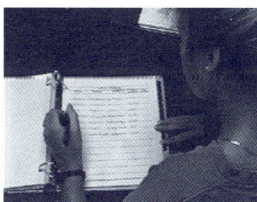

The Chemical Inventory must be accurate and thorough because it determines the remainder of your Hazard Communication Program. However, since training is based on the potential exposure for the specific chemicals each employee uses, there must also be an assessment of employee tasks. This assessment, discussed in Course #7, is the Chemical Exposure Determination and is similar to the Exposure Determination in Course #2. Each employee's tasks should be reviewed to determine the chemicals they use. Training for each employee is tailored to the chemicals they actually use.

Each chemical your practice uses must be evaluated for its potential to cause adverse health effects and its ability to pose physical hazards, such as flammability. Any chemical found to be a suspected or confirmed carcinogen must be reported to employees as such.

The detailed inventory is merely a list of all chemicals used in the practice. Additional information, critical to the safe use of a chemical, is found on the SDS. One SDS is required for each chemical listed in the inventory. SDSs are kept in a central location, whether in a file or binder, that is accessible to all employees.

Where are the SDSs kept in your practice?

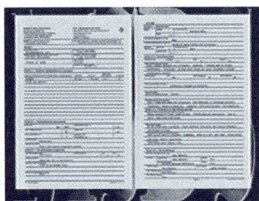

_____

An SDS is a technical fact sheet that describes the ingredients, hazards, and emergency procedures for a toxic product. Manufacturers and importers prepare an SDS for each hazardous product they produce or import, and distributors must also maintain an SDS for the products they distribute. Your employer must, in turn, provide the SDS to you, or to your healthcare provider, if necessary. This process of generating and disseminating information is called "downstream flow of information" and is the method of passing the information from producers of chemicals to you.

Chemical Manufacturers/Importers

- Determine the hazards of each product

Chemical Manufacturers/Importers & Distributors

- Communicate the hazard information and associated protective measures to customers through labels and SDSs

Employers

- Identify and list hazardous chemicals in their workplace
- Obtain SDSs and labels for each hazardous chemical
- Develop and implement a written Hazard Communication Program, including labels, SDSs, and employee training that is based on the list of chemicals, SDSs, and label information
- Communicate hazard information to employees through labels, SDSs, and formal training programs

Regarding the revised HCS and how it relates to the Safety Data Sheet (SDS), OSHA believes that use of a consistent format will improve the effectiveness of SDSs by making information easier for the reader to find, regardless of the supplier of the SDS. Because the newer 16-section format is accepted by consensus as the most appropriate format, OSHA no longer endorses that Form 174 be used for the preparation of SDSs. Use of form 174, however, is still acceptable under the HCS if it is completed correctly. The sample SDS Sheet on the following page is form 174.

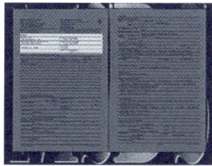

1 **Product or chemical identity used on the label:** The same as appears on the Chemical Inventory. Formal chemical names are useful if a single chemical is involved; mixtures may not have a formal name.

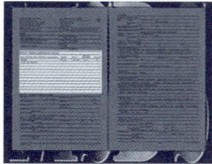

2 **Name, address, and phone number for hazard and emergency information**

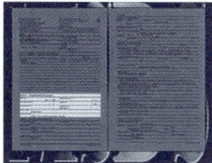

3 **Date of SDS preparation**

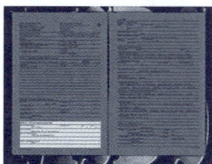

4 **Chemical and common names of hazardous ingredients:** Applies to mixtures, the list of ingredients that constitute the known hazard of the mixture, or the list of ingredients that have health effects and that comprise 1% or more of the mixture, except for carcinogens that comprise 0.1% or more of the mixture. Also included is a Chemical Abstracts Service (CAS) number which identifies a chemical with certainty—there is only one number per chemical, although a chemical may have several product names.

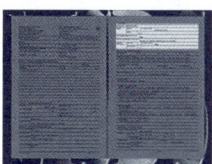

5 **OSHA Permissible Exposure Limit (PEL), American Conference of Governmental Industrial Hygienists (ACGIH) Threshold Limit Value (TLV), and other applicable limits:** TLVs are recommendations and not legally enforceable, OSHA PEL is the maximum amount of a substance legally allowed in workplace air. These values may be similar.

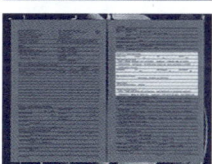

6 **Physical and chemical characteristics:** Properties of the product such as boiling point, flash point, vapor pressure and density, solubility, appearance, odor, specific gravity, melting point and evaporation rate.

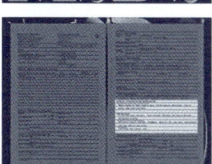

7 **Physical hazards, including the potential for fire, explosion and reactivity**

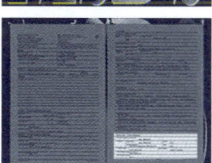

8 **Primary routes of entry into the body, such as inhalation, ingestion, or skin absorption**

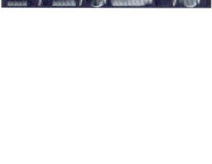

9 **Acute and chronic health hazards, including signs and symptoms of exposure and medical conditions aggravated by exposure**

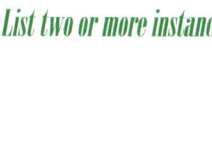

10 **Carcinogenic hazard:** National Toxicology Program (NTP) Annual Report on Carcinogens, International Agency for Research on Cancer (IARC) Monographs, or chemicals regulated by OSHA. Not required unless a carcinogen.

11 **Emergency and first aid procedures**

12 **Precautions for safe handling and use including hygienic practices, repair and maintenance, protective measures, and spill/leak cleanup**

13 **Exposure control measures such as Engineering and Work Practice Controls, and PPE**

An SDS contains information that is very technical. It is the responsibility of your employer to help you understand each SDS so that the appropriate handling and PPE may be used to reduce the risk of a chemical exposure. Everyone should be prepared for potential emergency situations.

List two or more instances when you would need to use an SDS.

_____

_____

Safety Data Sheet

May be used to comply with
OSHA's Hazard Communication Standard.
29 CFR 1910.1200. Standard must be
consulted for specific requirements.

U.S. Department of Labor

Occupational Safety and Health Administration
(Non-Mandatory Form)
Form Approved
OMB No. 1218-0072

IDENTITY *(As Used on Label and List)* ①

Note: Blank spaces are not permitted. If any item is not applicable, or no information is available, the space must be marked to indicate that.

Section I

Manufacturer's Name ②	Emergency Telephone Number
Address *(Number, Street, City, and ZIP Code)*	Telephone Number for Information
	Date Prepared ③
	Signature of Preparer *(optional)*

Section II -- Hazardous Ingredients/Identity Information

Hazardous Components (Specific Chemical Identity; Common Name(s))	OSHA PEL	ACGIH TLV	Other Limits Recommended	% *(optional)*
④		⑤		

Section III -- Physical/Chemical Characteristics

Boiling Point		Specific Gravity ($H_2O = 1$)	
Vapor Pressure (mm Hg) ⑥		Melting Point	
Vapor Density (AIR = 1)		Evaporation Rate (Butyl Acetate = 1)	
Solubility in Water			
Appearance and Odor			

Section IV - Fire and Explosion Hazard Data

Flash Point (Method Used) ⑥	Flammable Limits	LEL	UEL
Extinguishing Media ⑦			
Special Fire Fighting Procedures			
Unusual Fire and Explosion Hazards			

Section V -- Reactivity Data

Stability	Unstable		Conditions to Avoid
	Stable		

Incompatibility *(Materials to Avoid)*   **7**

Hazardous Decomposition or By-products

Hazardous Polymerization	May Occur		Conditions to Avoid
	Will Not Occur		

Section VI -- Health Hazard Data

Route(s) of Entry:	Inhalation? **8**	Skin?	Ingestion?

Health Hazards *(Acute and Chronic)*

9

Carcinogenicity: **10**	NTP?	IARC Monographs?	OSHA Regulated?

Signs and Symptoms of Exposure   **9**

Medical Conditions: Generally Aggravated by Exposure

Emergency and First Aid Procedures   **11**

Section VI -- Precautions for Safe Handling and Use

Steps to Be Taken in Case Material Is Released or Spilled

12

Waste Disposal Method

Precautions to Be Taken in Handling and Storing

Other Precautions

Section VIII -- Control Measures

Respiratory Protection *(Specify Type)*   **13**

Ventilation	Local Exhaust		Special
	Mechanical *(General)*		Other

Protective Gloves	Eye Protection

Other Protective Clothing or Equipment

Work/Hygienic Practices   **12**

- **If an SDS for any chemical is missing, has no date, is old, or is illegible, ask your distributor or the manufacturer to supply a new one. Each SDS should be dated when it is received. If after requesting an SDS you fail to receive one, your Infection Control Coordinator or Safety Officer should contact OSHA and inform them. The process of maintaining a full and complete SDS file need not be a difficult one.**

- **SDSs for products replaced or no longer used should not be thrown out. Products can change their chemical composition and you or other employees may wish to know the ingredients of a product at a later date. These SDSs should be removed from the SDS binder and stored in a different file with the older chemical lists.**

- **Some dental distributors use a computer-based ordering system that automatically sends an SDS any time a chemical is ordered for the first time. Ask your distributor if this service is available.**

Consumer Product Exemptions

If a product is excluded under the Consumer Products Exemption Category from the Hazard Communication Standard, an SDS is not required. Your employer must be able to prove, however, that the product is used in the same fashion and frequency as it would be for normal consumer use.

Hazard Abatement

Hazard Abatement is the next step in your Hazard Communication Program. The goal of Hazard Abatement is to avoid hazards or potential hazards. Container labels, workplace signs, and training are used to communicate the hazards of the toxic substances and the established procedures used to minimize your risk.

Container Labeling

In the U.S., OSHA requires that all chemical manufacturers, importers, and distributors be sure that containers of hazardous chemicals both in the workplace and when being disposed are labeled, tagged or marked with the full name of chemical, appropriate hazard warnings, and the name and address of the manufacturer or other responsible party.

In the workplace, each container should be labeled, tagged, or marked with the identity of hazardous chemicals contained therein, and must show hazard warnings appropriate for employee protection. The hazard warning can be any type of message (words, pictures, or symbols) that convey the hazards of the chemical(s) in the container. Labels must be legible, in English (plus other languages, if desired), and prominently displayed.

Because the manufacturer or distributor is required to provide products with appropriate warnings on the label, it is not necessary to apply a new label unless the product is removed from the original container.

The labeling of the original container of a product is the responsibility of the manufacturer, distributor, or importer and it is not necessary to apply a new label unless the product is removed form the original container. The Infection Control Coordinator or Safety Officer, or another designated person, should check the label to see if it meets labeling requirements discussed earlier in this course under the revised 2012 Hazard Communication Standard.

Labels must contain:

- **Appropriate hazard warnings**
- **Identification of the chemical**
- **Manufacturer's name and address**

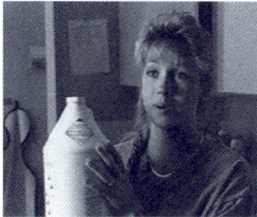

Products that are subject to EPA regulations (the Federal Insecticide, Fungicide, and Rodenticide Act: disinfectants) and FDA regulations (food, food additives, color additives, drugs, or medical devices) must be labeled by the manufacturer according to the respective agency's regulations. There is no need to relabel these containers, but you may find that one standard label, applied by your practice, adds useful information when handling the chemical. Labels should serve as an immediate visual warning that a hazard may be present.

A practice-specific and practice-applied label may do this best. Different formats of labels are available from many sources and you can even use a blank label that you can complete with the appropriate information. Your practice should use a label that is easy to understand by everyone. Information that may be useful on a practice-applied label include:

- **PPE required for safe use**
- **Routes of entry**
- **Emergency Actions**
- **Product Number, if numerical system is used for Chemical Inventories and SDSs**

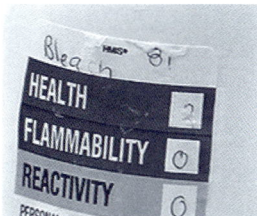

If any chemical is transferred to another container, that new, or secondary container must be labeled. The label on the secondary container must contain the same information required for the label on the original container. This is easily accomplished by obtaining a duplicate copy of the label or by filling in a blank label.

Note:

If you are supplied a sample product by a salesperson, the container must be labeled. In addition, the sales person should supply an SDS and if the product is to be used and employees exposed, the product should be entered into the Chemical Inventory.

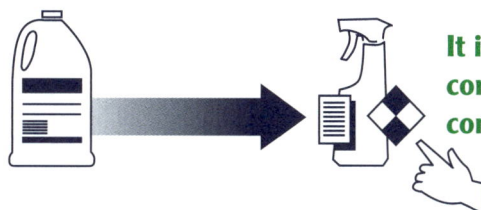

It is necessary to label a bottle correctly after filling it from another container.

Secondary Labeling Exemption

An exemption to the secondary labeling rule is the one that applies to daily use. If, for example, you are pouring an iodophor from a large bottle to a smaller container, and *you are the only person* who will be using the smaller container during the day and it will remain under your control before it is emptied or disposed, the secondary bottle does not need to be labeled. If that smaller bottle is shared with anyone, it must be appropriately labeled. Always label secondary containers to avoid chemical mishaps.

Signs

Another method of transmitting hazard information is through signs in the workplace. Examples include: a sign outside of a closed cabinet stating what is inside, an Eyewash Station sign, and posters that explain labeling or portions of your Hazard Communication Program. Signs and posters are available from many sources or you can make your own.

Employee Training

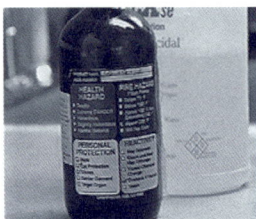

Employee training for chemical hazards is required and ensures safe handling of chemicals, informs you of the potential hazards associated with chemicals you use, assists in an emergency, and is required. Training is specific for each chemical and hazard that chemical presents.

Follow-up is necessary to determine if training was successful and if retraining is necessary for some employees. As an alternative, regular training may be used to ensure that all employees handle chemicals properly. Training is also required when you have a change in your duties that may expose you to different chemicals, or any time a new chemical that you may use is introduced in the practice.

If there is a chemical used in the practice by others that you will never use or come in contact with, you do not need to be trained for that particular chemical. To ease the management of training, all employees may be trained the same way for all chemicals in use. This practice is advisable because you may occasionally have to use different chemicals, and the additional training would then be required.

Training Requirements

At a minimum, a Hazard Communication Training Program must include:

- **Information on the Hazard Communication Standard, its requirements, and any other relevant state regulations.**
- **Location of the written Hazard Communication Program, Chemical Inventory and the SDSs.**
- **An overview of the hazards of chemicals in the work area.**
- **Where chemicals are located and how they are stored.**
- **The location of the SDSs, and how to read and interpret them. You should also receive information on how to use the information provided.**
- **An explanation of how the Hazard Communication Program is implemented in the office.**

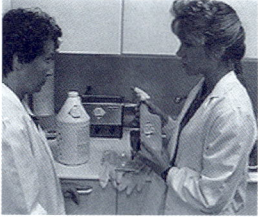

Training for specific chemicals must be provided in your practice by your employer, the Infection Control Coordinator or Safety Officer, or another designated person. It is impossible to train you, in the context of this course, for all possible chemicals that may be used in dentistry. To train for each specific chemical, you should understand its proper use and control procedures used in your practice when handling that particular chemical. Training for specific chemicals includes:

- **Measures you can take to protect yourself from the potential hazards, including:**
  - The use of appropriate PPE
  - Specific procedures, and Work Practice and Engineering Controls determined by your employer and/or recommended by the manufacturer of the chemical
- **Methods and observations, such as visual appearance or smell, that you can use to detect the presence of a hazardous chemical**
- **Measures to be taken in the event of a chemical exposure**

Tips & Hints

- **To train for smell detection, place a small amount of the chemical in an open container and smell it—carefully. Prior to doing this, check the chemical's SDS to be certain that smelling, even a small whiff, is not dangerous.**

or: **The smells of a dental office may be non-distinct. Employees should help each other distinguish what smells belong to which chemicals, especially the more hazardous ones. In this way, everyone should be able to detect the presence of a chemical, even by smell.**

List four chemicals you use on a regular basis and fill out the information below.

	Chemical	List all PPE Used	Specific Procedures (Work Practice and Engineering Controls)
Example:	Iodophor Disinfectant	Clinic Attire, Utility Gloves, Mask, Eyewear	- Use a funnel when transferring into another container, - Spray/Wipe/Spray when using.
❶			
❷			
❸			
❹			

What would you do if you spilled a chemical or splashed some on yourself or someone else? For spills, the initial step is to reduce the spill or minimize the area the spill affects. For an exposure incident, you would first minimize the exposure injury by applying immediate and appropriate first aid. These actions start the process of Hazard Containment.

Foreseeable Emergencies

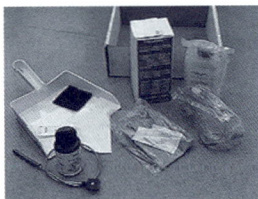

Employers must be prepared for any foreseeable emergency that may occur when working with hazardous substances. According to OSHA, foreseeable emergencies include "any potential occurrence such as, but not limited to, equipment failure, rupture of containers, or failure of control equipment which could result in an uncontrolled release of a hazardous chemical into the workplace."

The information describing how to deal with emergencies is included in each chemical's SDS. For spills, your response can range from simply vacuuming a powder, to neutralizing a chemical with another substance, to evacuation of the area and the need for emergency respirators and PPE. The SDS must be consulted if you are not totally familiar with the proper cleanup procedure. For most hazardous substances, it is advisable to review the procedure to be prepared in the event of an emergency.

Tips & Hints

- **There are emergency spill products available for spills in the workplace. Some manufacturers combine products into Emergency Spill Kits, which are designed to handle both blood and chemical spills.**

Chemical Exposures

Follow-up to a chemical exposure is a two-step process. First, you must recognize that you or someone else has been or is being exposed. Second, you must treat the exposed person with first aid. If a chemical is splashed on someone, it is usually evident that an Exposure Incident has occurred. But what about an inhalation of chemical vapor or gas? Part of your chemical-specific training is to be able to recognize the signs and symptoms that may occur to yourself or someone else following an exposure. This information is also in each chemical's SDS.

Emergency Medical Procedures

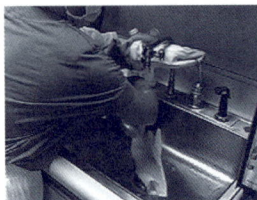

If exposed to a chemical, follow the emergency procedures found on the SDS. For example, if a chemical is ingested, one SDS may indicate that the proper first aid is to induce vomiting while others will say not to induce vomiting, but to administer milk or other liquids orally. The response is dictated by the specific chemical involved. If you are unsure of the response, call the manufacturer using the number on the SDS, or call your local poison control center.

In Course #2, we discussed emergency procedures for various exposure incidents. To review the procedure for a chemical exposure incident, you would:

1. **Treat the injury as appropriate.**

   For most chemical splashes onto yourself or another person, you would immediately flush the area with water for a minimum of 10-15 minutes. This includes splashes into your eyes. For this reason, every dental office must have an eyewash station and everyone should know where it is, be able to reach it, and be trained how to use the station properly.

2. **Immediately notify the Infection Control Coordinator or Safety Officer or senior employee.**

   This step is basically a call for help. After the initial first aid, you must get someone else involved to assist in getting you or the employee you are assisting to proper medical treatment.

3. **Get the Infection Control/Exposure Control Plan, and follow Tab "B" for your practice's Chemical Postexposure Management Plan.**

   This plan, developed in advance of any exposure incident, is a step-by-step procedure to follow when emergencies occur. If you are not familiar with your practice's Postexposure Management Plans, locate the Exposure Control Manual and review the plans at this time.

Tips & Hints

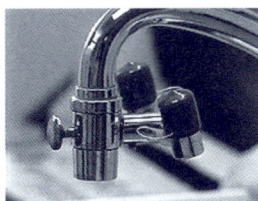

- **All employees must be trained in the proper use of the eyewash station. One suggested method of additional training is to blindfold each employee, and then have them find their way to the eyewash station and turn the water on while blindfolded. This will ensure that even if you are left alone in the office, you can find and use the eyewash station in the event of a chemical splash.**

- **When using an eyewash station, turn your head to the side and let the water run down over your eyes. The use of too much pressure directly into the eyes may cause additional injury.**

- **Some chemicals' SDSs may state a different first step in treatment. Flushing with water may be inappropriate. As these are unusual, you may want to note which of these chemicals, if any, are used in your practice. The chemical's label should indicate this difference.**

- **As discussed previously, your first aid kit should include the necessary items for chemical exposures of the type that may happen with the chemicals used in your office.**

- **Your emergency procedures should contain plans in the event that a chemical exposure is so extensive that the use of an eyewash station or sink is not sufficient. If someone spills a bottle of chemicals on themselves, is there a shower facility nearby or other means to flush the affected area?**

Using the same four chemicals you use on a regular basis (pg. 17), fill out the information below.

CHEMICAL	SPILL PROCEDURE	EMERGENCY PROCEDURE FOR SPLASH TO:		
		Eyes	Skin	Mouth/Nose
Example: Iodophor Disinfectant	Wipe with toweling	Use eyewash station to flush for 5-10 minutes	Flush skin for 5-10 minutes	Flush areas for 5-10 minutes
❶				
❷				
❸				
❹				

Checklist for Compliance & Safety

Your employer has a responsibility to inform you of the hazards in the workplace. Specifically for chemical hazards, your employer must:

1. **Obtain a copy of the Hazard Communication Standard; read and understand the requirements**
2. **Assign responsibility for tasks**
3. **Write a Hazard Communication Program**
4. **Develop a Chemical Inventory**
5. **Gather the SDSs for the chemicals in use and make available to employees**
6. **Label containers and post any necessary signs**
7. **Train employees prior to initial use of any chemical and retrain as necessary**
8. **Establish procedures to maintain a current hazard control program and to evaluate the program's effectiveness**
9. **Have all necessary PPE available**
10. **Have appropriate first aid for emergencies that may occur with the chemicals known to be present in the practice**

As an employee you also have responsibilities for your practice's Hazard Communication Program. Specifically you must know where to find:

1. **The written Hazard Communication Program**
2. **The Chemical Inventory**
3. **The SDS file/binder**
4. **The eyewash station**
5. **The first aid kit(s)**
6. **Appropriate PPE and Engineering Controls**

In addition you must be trained:

1. **How to use the written Hazard Communication Program and the Chemical Inventory**
2. **How to read an SDS for the appropriate information**
3. **How to read your practice's container labels**
4. **How to detect chemical spills or accidents,** including signs and symptoms or reactions to an exposure.
5. **How to protect yourself while working with chemicals,** including the appropriate PPE for each chemical, and procedures (Work Practice and Engineering Controls) for handling all chemicals, as outlined in the SDS and on the label.
6. **To understand what procedures to follow in the case of a chemical exposure incident**

It is important to understand and follow the OSHA regulations regarding chemical safety and hazard management and to also follow any specific state Right-To-Know Laws.

Discussion

Discuss with your Infection Control Coordinator or Safety Officer your practice's hazard communication program including how to access the chemical inventory and safety data sheets.

Objectives

Upon completion of this course on medical waste disposal, you will be able to:

1. Compare and contrast the various classifications of waste in the oral health-care setting.

2. Explain four steps in managing regulated waste.

3. Differentiate between medical waste, hazardous waste and toxic waste

4. Provide an example for each of the following categories of waste: regulated waste (chemical hazardous, biohazardous), and non-regulated waste (non-hazardous/household).

5. Explain the role of Personal Protective Equipment (PPE) in handling medical waste.

Focus

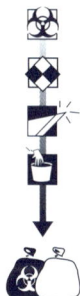

A dental practice deals with materials that are hazardous due to their infectious, toxic, or physical injury potential. To help prevent injury and maintain a safe work environment, there are established procedures and selected equipment that may minimize your risk.

Dental practices also generate waste that is either general waste or regulated waste. Regulated waste may be infectious, hazardous, toxic, or otherwise dangerous. A generator of hazardous waste is responsible for safe handling, storage, transportation, and disposal of this waste.

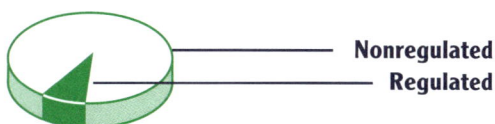

Nonregulated — Regulated

Medical Waste Tracking Act

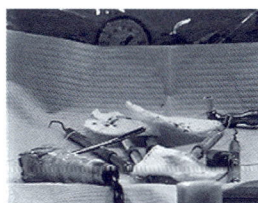

Medical waste was not always regulated. In response to public attention resulting from several well-publicized events in 1987, the Medical Waste Tracking Act (MWTA) was signed in 1988. This Act created a pilot program to determine if the proper disposal of medical waste could be guaranteed under federal law. Laws and regulations concerning other hazardous waste were already in effect. There is, however, some controversy about the actual hazard associated with medical (infectious) waste. The CDC, in the preamble to the MWTA, stated that "...there is no epidemiologic evidence to suggest that most hospital waste is any more infectious than residential waste, nor is there evidence of disease transmission as the result of improper waste disposal."

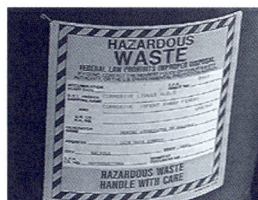

After regulated waste leaves your practice, the transport and ultimate disposal of hazardous waste is regulated by the federal EPA as well as various state and local agencies. Your practice remains responsible for the hazardous waste it generates until it is destroyed or rendered nonhazardous. This concept is called "cradle to grave" liability and means that even after waste leaves your practice, any cleanup for any damage it may cause is the responsibility of the generator (your practice). The proper handling and disposal of waste is something that cannot be taken lightly.

The handling, storage, and disposal of waste depends entirely on what the waste is, and the disposal of some waste can be expensive. Therefore, to comply with regulations *and* to minimize disposal costs, waste should be segregated, when generated, according to its type. For example, when processing an operatory, the waste is segregated into different containers at that time. But what waste goes in which container?

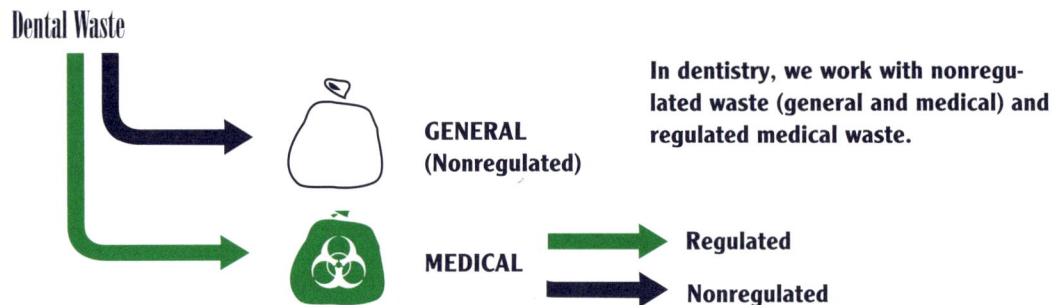

Dental Waste

GENERAL
(Nonregulated)

MEDICAL

Regulated

Nonregulated

In dentistry, we work with nonregulated waste (general and medical) and regulated medical waste.

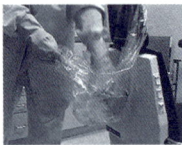

General Waste

General waste is all nonhazardous, nonregulated waste. Examples include waste generated by a front desk employee or waste from an employee lunch.

Medical Waste

Any general waste that is generated in diagnosis or treatment is considered medical waste. Medical waste can either be regulated or nonregulated. Nonregulated medical waste may be the same as general waste and includes gloves, masks, disposable gowns, lightly soiled gauze or cotton rolls, and environmental barriers. According to the EPA, waste generated by healthcare providers in private homes is considered household waste.

Regulated Waste

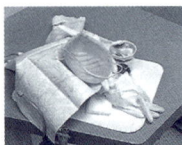

Regulated waste carries a substantial risk of causing infection during handling and disposal. Examples include gauze saturated with blood, extracted teeth, surgically removed hard and soft tissues, and contaminated sharp items such as needles, scalpel blades, and wires. Be sure to review state and local laws for specific handling and disposal requirements.

Medical Waste Determination

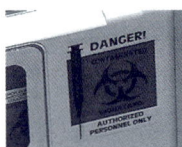

Regulated medical waste is contaminated waste that exhibits specific characteristics. There are three types of regulated medical waste in most dental practices:

1. **Blood and blood-saturated materials:** Gauze, cotton rolls, etc.
2. **Pathological waste:** Tissue and extracted teeth. However, if teeth contain amalgam, other concerns apply.
3. **Sharps:** Any sharp object used for patient care.

The determination of a regulated medical waste is made without regard to the patient's disease status. Remember that the concept of Standard Precautions states that all patients are treated in a similar manner, whether their infectious status is known or not known.

The strict definition of hazardous waste is any waste that poses a risk or peril to humans or the environment. Medical waste is also hazardous, and sometimes considered biohazardous waste. Hazardous waste does not have to be infectious and most often, hazardous waste refers to hazardous and toxic chemicals and materials.

Some items, such as extracted teeth with amalgam, may be both regulated hazardous and medical waste. After disinfection, teeth with amalgam are considered only hazardous waste and may be disposed with scrap amalgam.

Note:

For this course, we will refer to all chemical waste as hazardous waste. Hazardous waste can be either solid (lead foil, scrap amalgam), or liquid (spent fixer).

Toxic Waste

Toxic waste is any waste capable of having a poisonous effect. Toxic waste is a subset of hazardous waste and therefore, all toxic waste is hazardous waste, but not all hazardous waste is toxic waste.

Compliance Agencies

Dental waste comes under the jurisdiction of different agencies depending on the waste generated and where your practice is located. Inside the office, OSHA regulations on handling waste take precedence. The transportation and disposal of waste is the responsibility of the federal EPA and/or local and state regulatory agencies.

Many of the regulations that control the disposal of waste are at a state level. In addition, transporters of regulated waste may be regulated by the Department of Transportation (DOT) or state agencies. The CDC and professional organizations also make recommendations regarding the safe disposal of waste.

Note:

In many cases, state and local laws are more stringent than federal mandates and, in every case, the most stringent laws apply.

The management of regulated waste should not be difficult. Generally, it can be divided into four steps:

1. **Handling, Segregating, and Storing:** Activities in the practice for storage, prior to transportation and disposal.
2. **Labeling:** Regulated waste must be labeled prior to transporting to the disposal site.
3. **Disposing:** The step in which waste is either rendered nonhazardous or destroyed.
4. **Record Keeping:** Documenting the disposal or treatment process for waste generated by your practice. This ensures that the waste ends up where it is supposed to and your practice can verify the disposal.

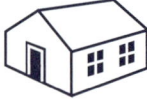

One of the main components of the Resource Conservation and Recovery Act (RCRA) is that it allows states and localities to adopt and enforce their own laws – some of which may be more stringent than federal laws. In this course we will discuss these federal laws, but every practice should contact its state Environmental Protection Agency (EPA) or state Department of Environmental Protection (DEP) for any variation or more stringent interpretation of what may be required.

Generators of waste must follow state regulations for the transportation and disposal of their waste depending on the amount of waste they produce. The more a generator produces, the stricter the guidelines that must be followed. To determine your practice's generator classification, you must assess the amount of waste generated in each category of regulated waste: medical and hazardous. The following are examples (the actual amounts of waste per classification and the names of each classification vary from state to state):

Medical Waste

- **Very-Small-Quantity Generator:** Practices that generate less than 50 pounds of regulated medical waste per month. In most states, only infectious waste is considered regulated medical waste. These generators are not exempt from proper packaging, labeling, and transport of their waste. Most dental practices are in this category. (Note: regulations vary and medical waste is measured in pounds while hazardous waste is measured in kilograms.)

Hazardous Waste

- **Conditionally Exempt Small-Quantity Generator:** Practices that generate less than 100 kilograms of regulated hazardous waste, or not more than 1 kilogram of acutely hazardous waste, per month.

- **Small-Quantity Generator:** Practices that generate between 100 and 1,000 kilograms of regulated hazardous waste per month.

- **Large-Quantity Generators:** Practices that generate 1,000 kilograms or more of regulated hazardous waste, or more than 1 kilogram of acutely hazardous waste per month.

Note:

Waste regulations may vary among states and local communities. Always refer to your local and state laws concerning waste disposal.

What is the classification of your practice?

Medical: _____

Hazardous: _____

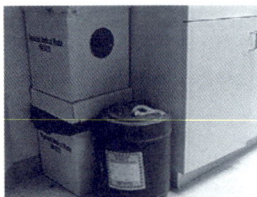

For all of the categories above, the amounts stated include how much is accumulated on the premises per month. Your practice, therefore, must package and transport regulated waste on a schedule that keeps the amount on the premises below the threshold limit for the next category. For most practices, transporting its own waste on a monthly basis may be adequate.

Generators of waste are subject to additional requirements, including one or more of the following:

Registration: Generators of regulated waste usually must register with a state agency for each type of regulated waste.

License or Permit: Some states may require a generator to receive a license or I.D. number.

Transport License: Transporters may be required to receive a special license from the federal DOT or the state DOT prior to transporting waste. The same may hold true for practices transporting their own waste.

Registrations and licenses generally require an application process with the appropriate state agency and some states perform a site inspection.

Handling of Waste

The Bloodborne Pathogens Standard and the Hazard Communication Standard, as well as other more general OSHA regulations, govern how waste is managed in dental practices. OSHA states that the "disposal of all regulated waste shall be in accordance with applicable regulations of the United States..." Their concern is for the safety of employees handling waste in the office, not the subsequent transportation and disposal.

As regulations for waste disposal are waste-specific, it is most efficient and cost-effective to segregate waste when and where it is created. This means that you need a separate storage container for each method of disposal. For most states, there are four types of waste that need to be segregated:

1. Hazardous Waste

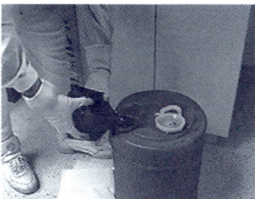

This is any waste that contains a hazardous chemical or material, even if it is also infectious. Examples include spent fixer, extracted teeth *with* amalgam, and lead foil from radiographs. Hazardous waste must be segregated according to the type of waste and disposal method. For example:

- **Spent fixer is placed into a labeled hazardous chemical container.**
- **Lead foil from radiographic film is placed into a lead foil container at the place where radiographs are processed.**
- **Extracted teeth containing amalgam should not be placed in a medical waste container intended for incineration as incineration can result in the release of toxic mercury vapors. For proper disposal consult state and local regulations. Some commercial hazardous waste haulers may be licensed for amalgam disposal. It is important to discuss the infectious as well as hazardous nature of teeth containing amalgam with the hazardous waste hauler to ensure that they are licensed both for regulated medical and toxic waste. Extracted teeth may be cleaned and placed in a leak-proof container, labeled as a biohazard, and in a liquid to keep them moist.**

2. Regulated Medical Waste

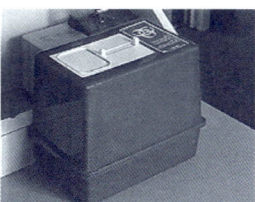

Dental regulated medical waste includes the three items mentioned earlier: blood-soaked items, extracted teeth (without amalgam), tissue, and contaminated sharps. Regulated medical waste is placed into two different containers: one for sharps and another for nonsharp infectious waste.

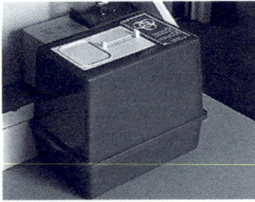

For sharps, including needles, broken instruments, glass ampules, wires, and teeth without amalgam, a sharps container is used. A sharps container is a closable, puncture-resistant container that is also leakproof on its sides and bottom and has a biohazard label or is color-coded red. During use, the container must be easily accessible and located as close as feasible to the area where sharps are used or anticipated to be found. It must also be upright at all times and disposed when 3/4 filled. Many companies and disposal firms offer containers that meet the above criteria.

Infectious: Nonsharp

Other, nonsharp regulated medical waste is placed in containers that are closeable, constructed to contain all contents and prevent leakage of fluids, labeled and/or color-coded, and closed prior to removal to prevent spillage. These containers must be kept apart from the general flow of traffic and refrigerated if necessary as pathogenic waste may decompose at room temperature. A common container is a 3-mil or thicker red plastic bag with a biohazard label on it.

All regulated medical waste must be marked with the international biohazard symbol and/or colored red. In addition, if the outside of the original container is contaminated or if leakage is possible, it must be placed into another container with the same criteria.

Recommendations for Extracted Teeth

- Dispose of extracted teeth as regulated medical waste unless returned to the patient.
- Do not dispose of extracted teeth containing amalgam in regulated medical waste intended for incineration.
- Clean and place extracted teeth in a leakproof container, labeled with a biohazard symbol, and maintain hydration for transport to educational institutions or a dental laboratory.
- Heat-sterilize teeth that do not contain amalgam before they are used for educational purposes.

3. Contaminated Waste

Contaminated waste, although not regulated for disposal, must be handled with gloves and should be placed into an appropriate container. To help identify contaminated waste receptacles, the following statement may be used: "Contains contaminated waste, do not handle without gloves." After isolating, the container can be handled without gloves and disposed as general waste, unless otherwise determined by state or local law.

4. General Waste

General waste is nonregulated, as there are currently no federal regulations regarding general waste. Any local regulations may only pertain to recycling issues.

Training

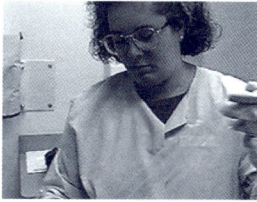

Employees should be trained in the handling of waste at the time of employment and at least annually thereafter. As part of the OSHA standards affecting dentistry, employees must be trained in the methods for handling and storing waste in the practice, the hazards associated with the waste, and any procedures to prevent or treat an exposure.

Where are the following stored in your practice, prior to transportation and disposal?

General Waste: _____

Contaminated Waste: _____

Infectious Waste: _____

Toxic Waste: _____

Preparing for Disposal

After segregation, disposal – where waste is either rendered nonhazardous or destroyed – is accomplished by following the steps for the specific type of waste for your location. The federal EPA has jurisdiction over the disposal, but careful attention must be paid to state and local regulations, which may be more stringent than the federal regulations.

All regulated dental waste must be disposed in a responsible manner. However, what constitutes "responsible" varies from state to state. For example, in some areas, liquid blood and blood products can be disposed via a sanitary sewer system. In other areas, typically rural ones, this type of medical waste must be transported and disposed of off-site.

Disposal Subcontractors

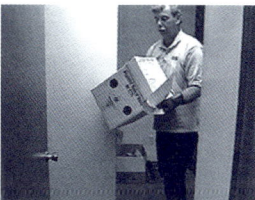

To facilitate proper transportation and disposal, your practice may subcontract with a licensed transporter, disposal, and/or recycling firm. Your employer is responsible for the waste until it is either rendered nonhazardous or destroyed, so choosing a disposal firm is an important decision. Disposal firms should be licensed and reputable. Use the same product selection criteria discussed in Course #6 and assemble as much information as possible about different firms that transport and dispose of dental waste, including how they guarantee appropriate disposal. The best resource for information may be other dental practices, local hospitals, or physicians.

Contracts between waste generators and disposal subcontractors should clearly identify responsibilities and liabilities associated with waste transport and disposal.

What is the name of the transport/disposal firm your practice uses for the following wastes?

Infectious: _____

Hazardous: _____

Labeling/Packaging

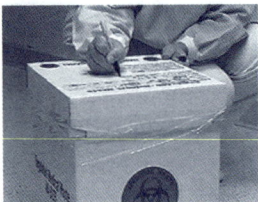

All regulated waste must be labeled, according to state law, in a way to ensure against removal of the label. The label may need to have the contents listed, as well as the name, address, and telephone number of the generator. In addition, all containers should be rigid, leak-resistant, impervious to moisture, strong enough so they will not be compromised during handling, and sealed to prevent leakage.

Note:

Disposal subcontractors may be able to supply your practice with necessary labels, forms, and/or containers to meet your state/local laws and regulations. However, you should verify their appropriateness with the proper regulatory agency.

Transporting

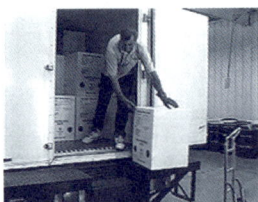

Waste is generally transported by a licensed hauler. The disposal firm your practice uses should have the appropriate licenses and permits to transport your waste. In some cases, a practice may want to transport its own waste either to a disposal facility or between sites in an effort to save on disposal costs by consolidating the regulated waste between different offices. Generally, a practice may transport only its own regulated waste, and any license or permit, if required, must accompany the waste. In some states, small medical practices are allowed to combine waste for transportation and disposal. Often this is a matter of submitting a plan to the regulating agency.

In addition to any limit on the amount of waste that is self-transported, waste must be packaged and labeled properly and incompatible wastes cannot be transported on the same shipment. Self-transportation may not be allowed in all states or may only be allowed for certain categories of generators.

To transport your own waste, you may have to register with the appropriate state agency a plan describing how and to where you will transport the waste. Even if the agency does not require a license, you should know what you would do in the event of an accident, emergency, or spill, and also who should be notified. Many states require immediate notification of state police.

Disposal

Every task you perform involving waste is preparing for its disposal. Waste must be segregated, placed in properly labeled containers, and transported to a disposal facility. All waste that is handled in-house must use proper techniques and record keeping.

Hazardous Waste

The most common types of hazardous waste generated by dental offices are spent fixer (which is a silver-bearing waste), scrap amalgam, and the lead foil packets from radiographic film.

Spent fixer can be disposed of by either hiring a transporter/recycler or by recycling the fixer in the practice, using a silver-recovery device or system. A common option is to choose a reputable firm to dispose of the spent fixer for the practice.

Scrap amalgam includes excess from restorative procedures, amalgam found in filter traps, and extracted teeth with amalgam. This waste should be kept in a liquid to keep it moist during transport in a appropriately labeled container for disposal as a hazardous waste or for recycling by authorized, licensed facilities. Amalgam, in any form, should never be heat-sterilized, as the heat from sterilization causes the release of toxic mercury vapors.

Lead foil packets should be segregated when processing radiographs. When the container is full, prepare for transport by closing the container and labeling as appropriate. Lead foil must be transported and disposed by a firm licensed to handle lead waste (which may require a special license). Some radiographic supply companies now offer to recycle the lead foil from their film.

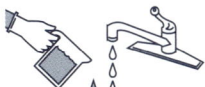

Hazardous Waste, Other: According to the EPA, it is acceptable to dispose of many chemicals down the drain into a sanitary sewer system with *copious* amounts of water. Local regulations may not allow this, especially if a local treatment plant cannot handle the chemicals. If your practice uses a sewer system, you should check to see if the system can handle the agents being disposed. Copious amounts of water stipulate a 1:30 dilution. That is, 1 part of chemical to 30 parts of water. If the chemical is a regulated hazardous waste, such as spent fixer, it cannot be disposed down the drain.

Name three chemicals used in your practice that can be safely disposed down the drain.

❶ _____

❷ _____

❸ _____

Regulated Medical Waste

After segregation, your practice should have two types of regulated medical waste, sharps and nonsharps. This waste must be transported and disposed by a licensed medical waste firm. Regulated infectious waste containers are available from dental distributors or waste disposal firms. To prepare for disposal, the containers must be sealed and labeled.

Rendering Your Waste Noninfectious

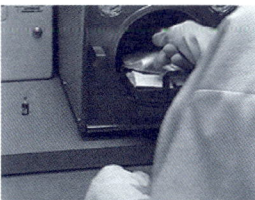

Regulated nonsharp medical waste may be treated in-house to render it noninfectious and then be disposed of with general waste. This may not be allowed in all states or locations. In areas where a practice *is* permitted to treat its own waste, there may be specific requirements that must be followed in the treatment process. For example, a practice may be permitted to sterilize medical waste to render it noninfectious prior to disposal. The same sterilizer used for instrument reprocessing may be used, but a separate cycle is usually required for the waste. In addition, there may be specific record keeping requirements.

If your practice treats its own infectious waste, you should follow your state or local requirements for disposal and consider the following:

- **Identify and follow state and local disposal regulations.**
- **Develop a written Standard Operating Procedure (SOP) for this procedure:** The SOP should describe, step-by-step, how to render waste noninfectious.
- **Package all waste prior to sterilization.**
- **Keep good written records:** Include who performed the sterilization, the method of sterilization, and the date. Also record the temperature and dwell time (the time at the appropriate temperature and/or pressure).
- **Biologic Monitor:** The only way to verify that each load of waste is successfully sterilized is to biologic monitor each load. The monitoring results are added to the written record.
- **Keep all records for three years,** unless otherwise indicated by local or state regulations.
- **Do not heat-sterilize teeth with amalgam or amalgam scrap:** The heat sterilization can cause amalgam to release mercury vapors into the air.

Exception: Sharps

An exception to the above, in terms of landfill disposal, is sharps. Even if sterilized to render noninfectious, sharps still present a physical hazard. There may be additional guidelines for sharps disposal other than to render them noninfectious.

Tip:

- **The best way to dispose of sharps is to place them into a sharps container at the point of use.**

Record Keeping

Keeping track of your dental waste involves monitoring activities both inside and outside the practice. Inside the practice, the amount of each type of waste is tracked to verify that your classification of waste generator is correct. There are additional record-keeping requirements if you treat your waste to render it noninfectious.

The EPA's "cradle to grave" rule holds waste generators responsible for proper disposal of their waste. A practice should carefully select a licensed hauler, *and* prepare and keep careful records regarding waste disposal to reduce its liability. Record keeping for the disposal of waste must meet the regulations for your state. The most critical record kept for waste transport is the waste manifest, which is a tracking document. The intent of a manifest is to identify the generator, the transporter, and the disposer, as well as the waste itself. A manifest may contain:

1. A description and quantity of the waste
2. The date
3. The type of container
4. The type of final disposal
5. The name, address and telephone number of the generator, the transporter and the disposer

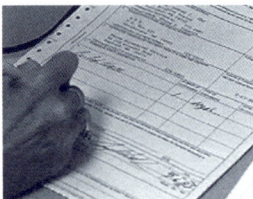

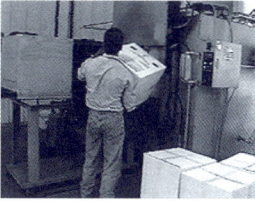

One person in the office should be designated to prepare, sign, and maintain the manifests. This person should also ensure that a copy of the manifest is returned from the disposal facility within 90 days (or the length of time your state allows) and filed with the pickup receipt. For each shipment of regulated waste, there will be two copies of the manifest filed – the copy proving pickup and the copy proving destruction.

Tips & Hints

If you do not receive a copy of the manifest back within 90 days, you should send a registered, return-receipt letter to the disposal facility and request the manifest. A copy of this letter should be kept on file with the copy of the manifest in question.

Manifest for Transportation

When preparing a manifest, the designated person will date, sign, and enter the address to which the waste is delivered. The transporter or agent of the transporter signs the manifest to indicate the waste was received and that there is agreement that the generator's instructions will be followed. The owner or agent of the owner of the disposal facility also signs the manifest and then, after disposal, returns the original to the generator.

Self-Transporting Record Keeping

A manifest may not be required if your practice self-transports waste. You must, however, keep a record of the type and quantity of waste, the date, the method of treatment and disposal. After the disposal facility receives the waste, be sure to obtain a proper receipt from the facility.

The record must show the method of disposal as well as other required information. All records for waste disposal, regardless of the manner of disposal, must be kept for three years.

Tips & Hints

Prior to self-transporting waste, check with both local and state regulations as some locations may require manifests.

Reducing Disposal Costs

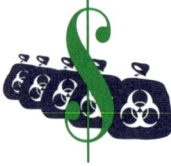

In an effort to streamline the medical waste disposal process, and to reduce costs as well as mistakes, your practice can "audit" waste production and disposal. A waste audit examines where and how dental waste is produced, and how it is contained, packaged and disposed. An audit may uncover ways to reduce waste, which in turn reduces the cost of packaging and disposal, and creates less stress on our environment.

The most economical and environmentally sound approach to reducing the disposal costs of waste is to reduce the amount of regulated waste you generate. If possible your practice should:

1. **Substitute nonhazardous products for hazardous.** When selecting products, avoid aerosol cans and use minimally hazardous chemicals.
2. **Modify your procedures without compromising treatment.**
3. **Segregate waste properly when generated. For example, contaminated waste should not be placed in infectious waste containers.**
4. **Recycle whenever possible.**
5. **Practice environmentally safe housekeeping.** Use reusable containers, etc.

The major issue in dental waste disposal is responsible disposal. The amount of medical waste generated by your office is dependent on patient load and work habits. Since regulations may change, a working relationship with your state's EPA/DEP and local organizations may be helpful. Up-to-date information will help ensure compliance with all government agencies (federal, state, and local).

Discussion

Discuss with your Infection Control Coordinator or Safety Officer the specific standard operating procedures for waste segregation and disposal.

Objectives

Upon completion of this course you will be able to:
1. Determine when updates should be made to an exposure control program
2. Identify four steps to create and maintain a safe work environment
3. Describe techniques that improve patient safety and project a safe and comfortable image.
4. Describe the basic elements of an effective exposure control program.

Focus

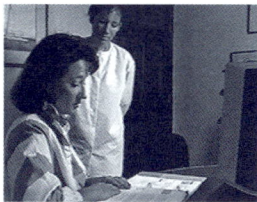

This is the last course in this series and you should now have a better understanding of your practice's Exposure Control Program. The challenge is to maintain an effective program over time. Updates need to be made as changes occur – a new employee may require a different type of glove, a new disinfectant that is more cost effective may come on the market, the ultrasonic cleaner you use may fail and you will have to purchase a new one.

How does a practice ensure that its Exposure
Control Program works and is successful?

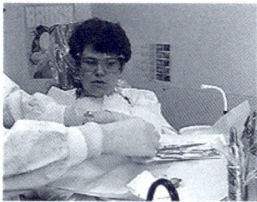

To work safely and be in compliance with evolving regulations, recommendations and standards of care, your practice may have instituted some changes. Most of the regulations that dictate your work practices are for the protection of you as an employee, but patients are also affected. Patients should be informed of your efforts to make them feel safe and comfortable.

How do you involve patients in your Exposure
Control Program?

Throughout this course series, elements of an effective Exposure Control Program have been discussed. For example, when discussing instrument reprocessing, the process of transporting, cleaning, sterilizing, and storing instruments was emphasized. Each step in this process was covered along with the types of equipment that may be used.

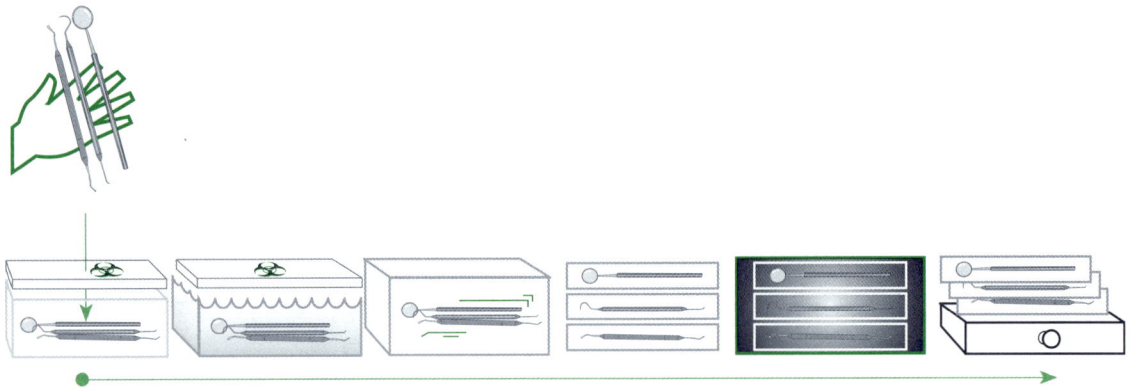

When reprocessing instruments, you must deal with infectious sharps and with hazardous chemicals and waste.

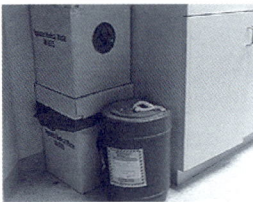

While topics were presented individually, they need to be integrated into a complete program for day-to-day practice. There are many different hazards in dentistry and there are a variety of procedures and products to manage the hazards. Following the example above, instruments are reprocessed using hazardous chemicals and waste is generated.

On a daily basis you must coordinate *all* the topics discussed in this series as they apply to your job and the tasks you perform.

How does it all fit together?

Program Evaluation: Reassessment

Throughout this course series, three major steps have been discussed for promoting a safe work environment: assessment, development, and implementation.

Assessment:

Assessment involves a review of a task or policy to determine what would be needed to create a safer environment. For example, you would remove any unnecessary items from the operatory prior to the development of a Standard Operating Procedure (SOP) for Operatory Processing.

Development:

Development involves the creation of an SOP that provides a method of how to perform a designated task. This standard set of procedures ensures that everyone in the practice performs various tasks in a similar manner.

Implementation:

An SOP is specific to a task such as operatory processing or instrument reprocessing. Anyone involved with a particular task must be aware of its SOP, be trained to the SOP, and use the SOP every time they perform (implement) that task.

The above three steps are crucial in the *establishment* of safe and effective practices. Their aim is to create workable and efficient procedures. But...

**How does a practice actually ensure that its
Exposure Control Program works and is successful?**

The answer is a fourth step *to maintain* a safe work environment.

Program Evaluation:

A written SOP is only as good as its implementation. Program Evaluation is necessary therefore, to continually reassess daily tasks in an effort to make the way you work as safe and up-to-date as possible. There should be an established routine evaluation of the infection control program, including evaluation of performance indicators, at an established frequency.

Who is responsible for monitoring the effectiveness of operatory processing in your practice?

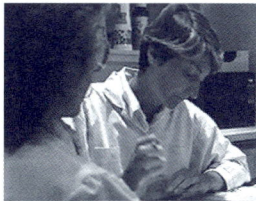

_____

_____

Program Evaluation should be both a formal and informal process. On a routine basis your employer and/or Infection Control Coordinator or Safety Officer should review the practice's policies and procedures at least once a year. In addition, policies and procedures must be reviewed as changes occur. Changes that necessitate reassessment may include new equipment, regulations, knowledge, or personnel.

Examples of methods for evaluating infection control programs

Appropriate immunization of dental healthcare personnel (DHCP):
- Conduct annual review of personnel records to ensure up-to-date immunizations.

Assessment of occupational exposures to infectious agents:
- Report occupational exposures to infectious agents. Document the steps that occurred around the exposure and plan how such exposure can be prevented in the future.

Comprehensive postexposure management plan and medical follow-up program after occupational exposures to infectious agents:
- Ensure the Postexposure Management Plan is clear, complete, and available at all times to all DHCP. All staff should understand the plan, which should include toll-free phone numbers for access to additional information.

Adherence to hand hygiene before and after patient care:
- Observe and document circumstances of appropriate or inappropriate handwashing. Review findings in a staff meeting.

Proper use of Personal Protective Equipment (PPE) to prevent occupational exposures to infectious agents:
- Observe and document the use of barrier precautions and careful handling of sharps. Review findings in a staff meeting.

Routine and appropriate sterilization of instruments using a biologic monitoring system:
- Monitor paper log of steam cycle and temperature strip with each sterilization load, and examine results of weekly biologic monitoring. Take appropriate action when failure of sterilization process is noted.

Evaluation and implementation of safer medical devices:
- Conduct an annual review of the Exposure Control Plan and consider new developments in safer medical devices.

Compliance with CDC's recommendation that routine dental treatment output water meets EPA regulatory standards for drinking water (i.e., $\leq$ 500 CFU/mL of heterotrophic water bacteria):
- Monitor dental water quality as recommended by the equipment manufacturer, using commercial self-contained test kits, or commercial water testing laboratories.

Proper handling and disposal of medical waste:
- Observe the safe disposal of regulated and non-regulated medical waste and take preventive measures if hazardous situations occur.

Tabulation of healthcare-associated infections:
- Assess the unscheduled return of patients after procedures and evaluate them for an infectious process. A trend might require formal evaluation.

In 2016, CDC published the *Summary of Infection Prevention Practices in Dental Settings: Basic Expectations for Safe Care.* This summary covers basic infection control expectations for safe dental care as described in the 2003 dental infection control guidelines and includes a checklist to evaluate infection control practices in the practice setting and among DHCP. More information about the summary and assessment tool are available through the CDC website at: www.cdc.gov/oralhealth/infectioncontrol or the OSAP website at: www.osap.org

Self-Evaluation

Employees should also review what they do on a routine basis. This "self-evaluation" is to ensure that you are working safely and according to a prescribed SOP. If there is an appropriate change to a procedure – maybe one that saves time or utilizes a different method – the corresponding SOP should also be changed.

If you notice anything that may improve an SOP, talk to your Infection Control Coordinator or Safety Officer or employer to officially modify the SOP rather than just changing the procedure for yourself. The change may also benefit others in the practice.

Each member of the practice should continually monitor practices, identify unsafe conditions, and help each other follow the practice's policies.

Example:

In one practice, the dental assistant responsible for operatory processing used a set of puncture-resistant/utility gloves that were kept in the instrument reprocessing area. Sometimes, and often when rushing, she would use the treatment gloves she wore during patient care to clean up because the utility gloves were "too far away." She noticed that there were several instances when she was almost stuck by a contaminated sharp.

After considering the situation thoroughly, she asked the Infection Control Coordinator to have a set of utility gloves placed in the operatory. This change was adopted and now she feels there is no excuse for not using her heavy duty gloves. As a result, she is working and feeling safer. NOTE: These gloves must be handled and stored as contaminated items, for example, they can be stored in the instrument transport container.

Part of this course's goal has been to create an atmosphere in which health and safety matters become second nature. While the primary role in dentistry is to treat patients, the safety of staff and patients is an integral component of providing care. This training will assist you in identifying and managing hazards in the workplace.

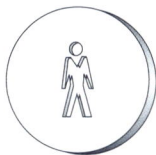

Your employer is ultimately responsible for ensuring safety in the workplace. There may be a designated Infection Control Coordinator or Safety Officer. However, you have a responsibility to participate in the practice's health and safety program: to comply with your practice's Exposure Control Program, to evaluate the program, and to offer feedback on its effectiveness. This role is crucial since you have the greatest familiarity with your tasks. If you notice any aspect of your daily tasks, or those of other employees, that may put you or others at risk, or if you notice ways to improve the efficiency of your practice, it is your responsibility to discuss this with the appropriate person in your practice.

Describe one task you perform that you feel should be improved. How could it be improved?

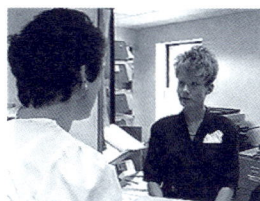

_____

_____

_____

_____

_____

_____

_____

Patient Awareness

How often do staff or patients ask questions about the practice's infection control policies or procedures? Patients may be more aware of potential risks that may *or may not* be present in dentistry. They may hear from friends how other dental practices operate and not fully understand why there may be differences between practices. They may even have read misleading articles or heard rumors of the "dangers" in dental treatment. A primary goal of dental infection control is to minimize risks to patients and staff.

How do you involve patients in your Exposure Control Program?

How a patient sees you and your practice may be different than the image you wish to project. A practice must assure staff and patients that health and safety are always priorities. From the moment a patient enters the practice, he or she should feel safe and comfortable. What you wear, where you wear it, what you say and how you say it, may be as important to a patient as your sterilization techniques or technical competency.

Everyone in the practice should be able to discuss all aspects of your Exposure Control Program with any patient. A patient may ask a nonclinical employee questions about sterilization, fearing that the same question may waste the time of clinical workers. Potential new patients may call a practice with questions about the infection control methods or techniques. For these and other reasons, it is advisable that everyone in the practice be trained to understand the Exposure Control Program and know when to refer questions to another appropriate person.

Techniques to improve patient safety and to project a safe and comfortable image include:

Proper clothing in the reception area.

When escorting a patient to or from the reception area, do not wear a mask, gloves, or eyewear (unless they are prescription glasses). By reserving the use of PPE to the operatories, it underscores the seriousness, usefulness, and patient-specific nature of PPE to patients.

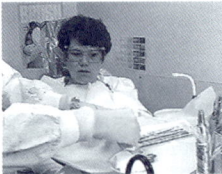

Open packaged sterilized instruments in front of the patient.

Open the package of sterile instruments and check the chemical indicator in front of the patient. This action demonstrates to the patient that the instruments have been properly reprocessed. It also provides an opportunity for the patient to ask questions about sterilization and the infection control process.

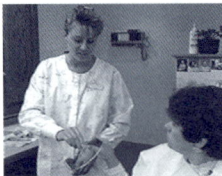

Offer patient eyewear.

Patient eyewear helps prevent traumatic injury to the eyes. If a patient does not have his/her own eyewear, a pair should be offered.

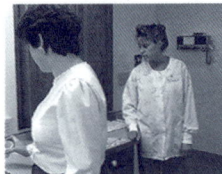

Offer a pretreatment mouthrinse.

This is a positive step for reducing the number of microorganisms in the mouth. It reduces the potential for microorganisms to be introduced into the bloodstream during invasive procedures. If a dental dam is indicated for treatment, discuss how this also helps reduce contaminated aerosols and protects the patient from swallowing or aspirating materials during dental treatment.

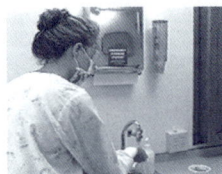

Wash your hands and don gloves in front of the patient

Performing these tasks in from of patients reassures them and demonstrates your concern for their safety.

These steps give the patient the opportunity to observe the practice's infection control techniques.

Listening to Patients

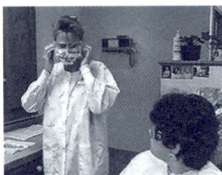

There is a tendency to approach children differently than adults in a clinical setting. Children may feel apprehensive about treatment and extra efforts may be made to help them feel more comfortable. You may use stickers or posters to put them at ease in addition to explaining everything you do.

Adults, however, may be taken for granted. In fact, adult patients may be even more apprehensive than younger patients. Part of this apprehension may translate into a desire to postpone or avoid dental treatment until absolutely necessary. All patients should be assured that health and safety are of genuine concern to the practice.

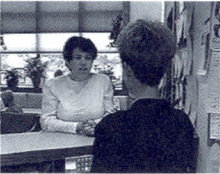

A difficult task in any busy practice is listening to the patient. If a patient asks a question, or makes a joke about barriers or sterilizing, they may be more concerned than it first appears. This is the time to respond as fully as possible. Do not answer in blanket statements such as "Oh, we sterilize everything." Rather you should answer their questions and offer specific information. Although you may need to answer the same question several times, it may be the first time a patient hears the answer, and for that patient, it needs to be done properly.

Note:

A patient may have heard or read that instruments should be sterilized in an autoclave and may ask you if you "autoclave" your instruments. They may even be expecting an answer of, "Yes we use an autoclave to sterilize your instruments." If in fact you have a chemiclave or dry heat sterilizer, you could answer, "No, we don't actually use an autoclave here." While the answer is accurate, it may not answer the patient's true question, or more importantly, relieve their anxiety.

Your answer should both directly answer the question and provide reasons why the answer may differ from the patient's expected answer. A suitable answer may be, "We don't use an autoclave, but we do use another sterilizing technique that is as effective. An autoclave works with steam under pressure while our sterilizer is a _____, which achieves the same results by _____. To ensure it works properly, we routinely check the equipment and monitor its effectiveness."

How would you explain Biologic Monitoring to a patient?

_____

_____

_____

_____

Patient Literature

Another way to assure patients your Exposure Control Program is effective is to provide literature in the reception area. In fact, it has been shown that practices that promote Exposure Control see an increase in new patients. Some topics for patient information may include:

- **Process of disease transmission**
- **Infection control specifics of the practice:**
  - **Type(s) of sterilizer used, and why all instruments are sterilized**
  - **Barriers used and why: What is cleaned and barrier-protected and what is cleaned and disinfected. As different practices may barrier-protect different surfaces, there may be confusion for some patients about your practice's barrier techniques.**
  - **Gloves, mask, eyewear, and gown used and why**
- **How the practice handles and disposes waste**

Indicate other techniques your practice may use to inform patients of your Exposure Control Program:

_____

_____

_____

If a patient asks you how they are protected in your practice, how would you answer?

_____

_____

_____

Basic Elements of an Effective Exposure Control Program

An Exposure Control Program has many parts, including written policies for Infection Control, Hazard Communication, and more.

How does it all fit together?

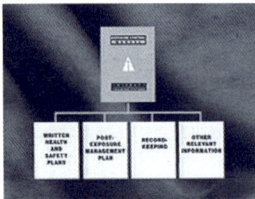

These policies represent your practice-specific Exposure Control Program. Policies or even compliance with government regulations, do not by themselves make for a safe practice. Developing an Exposure Control Program takes time. Each element must be developed and implemented, employees must be trained, and the entire Program must be evaluated to ensure that all plans and procedures work toward their intended goal. However, for a Program to be truly effective, everyone in your practice must believe in and buy into the process of Exposure Control and work together to achieve it.

Following are the basic elements of an effective Exposure Control Program:

A. Management Commitment and Leadership

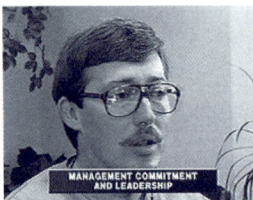

1. Goals established, issued, and communicated to all employees
This portion of a program is often implied in a dental practice. The use of this course is an example of your employer's desire to train employees. Practices in which the employer is not involved have a difficult time implementing any safety program and may have a dissatisfied staff.

2. Program review and revision
The written program must be reviewed annually and whenever there are changes in the practice. Revisions are necessary whenever there are changes in equipment, products, procedures, guidelines, or regulations.

3. Participation in safety meetings, evaluations
Your employer, or a designated person such as an Infection Control Coordinator or Safety Officer, takes the lead in this area. Safety meetings are held, as necessary, to discuss changes to your Program, to demonstrate new equipment

or techniques, to evaluate safer sharps or to review certain aspects of injuries or "near injuries." Evaluations are held routinely to assess the Program's effectiveness – this is the follow-up portion or "Program Evaluation" discussed earlier.

4. Adequate commitment of resources
Commitment of resources includes supplying appropriate PPE, Engineering Controls, and products necessary for safe practice.

5. Safety and health rules and procedures incorporated into site operations
SOPs are the actual methods used to perform tasks in a standardized manner expected of all employees.

6. Management observes safety and health rules
Everyone must follow established procedures – employers and Infection Control Coordinator or Safety Officers should set the example.

B. Assignment of Responsibility/Fixing Accountability

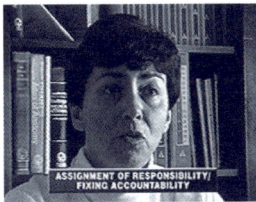

1. The safety and health designee on site is knowledgeable and accountable
The Infection Control Coordinator or Safety Officer is an important position for any safety program. It is this person's responsibility to train employees, to answer or know where to find answers to employees' questions, and to manage the implementation of the program. This individual should also constantly try to increase his/her knowledge of Exposure Control.

2. Employees understand their safety and health responsibilities
Employees are responsible for the tasks they perform and the health and safety associated with these. This responsibility must be taken seriously, including sharing concerns and suggestions with the Infection Control Coordinator or Safety Officer.

3. Employees adhere to safety and health rules and procedures
It is the responsibility of an employer to provide a safe worksite, but it is your responsibility to follow set procedures and work safely.

C. Identification and Control of Hazards

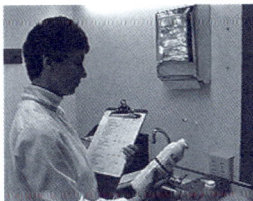

1. Periodic site safety and health evaluation program
Routinely assess the work site and procedures.

2. Preventative controls in place
Appropriately use PPE, Work Practice and Engineering Controls.

3. Action taken to address hazards
Ensure written plans, equipment and products, procedures, training, etc. are available. Also have manufacturers' instructions available.

4. Technical references available
Ensure equipment manuals, safety data sheets (SDSs), etc. are available.

5. Enforcement procedures by management
Specific policies should be established to address any staff refusals in following set procedures.

6. Modify work habits as necessary
Update work habits as changes occur.

D. Implementation of Training and Education into the Work Force

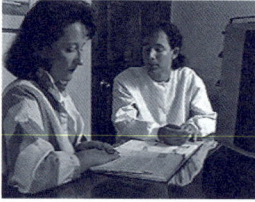

1. All employees receive basic training
This course is an example of basic training.

2. Specialized training is provided when indicated
For example, prior to using a hazardous chemical for the first time, employees must receive training specific to that chemical.

3. An employee training program is ongoing and effective
Some regulations require annual training, and some require training when necessary. Evaluation is used to determine if training is effective or if further training is required.

4. Employees are encouraged to develop safe work habits to reduce injuries
Work habit modification is a goal to reduce injuries.

E. Record Keeping and Hazard Analysis

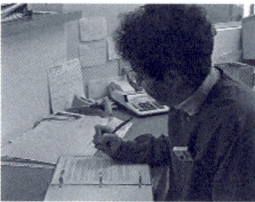

1. While federal OSHA record keeping forms are not required for dental offices, it is recommended that records of employee injuries/illnesses be maintained

2. The Infection Control Coordinator or Safety Officer performs accident investigations, determines causes, and proposes corrective action
If corrective action translates into a change of procedures, this must be incorporated into the written SOPs or plans.

3. Injuries, "near injuries" and illnesses are evaluated for trends and similar causes; corrective action is initiated as required
This is also part of the Program Evaluation step.

F. First Aid and Medical Assistance

A tailored program designed to meet the needs of the workplace.
Knowledge of methods to prevent illness and injury, and ways to manage injuries is essential. Your Postexposure Management Plan (the red tabs in the Exposure Control Manual) contains the procedures for managing injuries.

Knowledge, Attitude, Behavior

Congratulations on completing the OSAP Interact Infection Control & Safety Training System! This program has presented and reinforced the fundamentals of health and safety for dentistry. You should now have knowledge of the basic principles and procedures of infection control and safety including the CDC Guidelines and OSHA regulations. Your final challenge is to develop attitudes and behaviors consistent with the information presented in this program to protect you, other staff and your patients. Knowledge, attitude, and behavior work in unison to keep you and others safe and free from infectious diseases.

Be sure to retain your OSAP Interact workbook as a handy reference.

KNOWLEDGE · BEHAVIOR · ATTITUDE

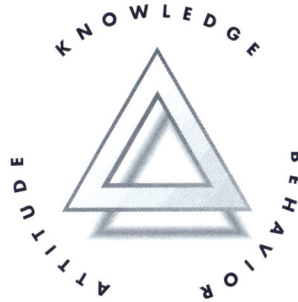

A safe workplace does not happen overnight.

With your enhanced knowledge, attitude,

and behavior, your practice will be a

safer and more desirable place

to practice dentistry.

Exposure Control Program Checklist

Your Infection Control Coordinator or Safety Officer has a checklist with blank spaces for practice-specific concerns. This list is not inclusive since this would not be practical. A checklist is affected by state and local regulations, practice-specific concerns, new guidelines and more. The following suggested list outlines many of the major points discussed in this course.

Review the following and think of how they relate to your practice's Exposure Control Program.

STAFF CONSIDERATIONS

- **Confidential Health Record**
- **Exposure Determination**
- **Routine Staff Education and Training**
- **Evaluation of Safer Sharps**
- **Hepatitis B Immunization/Vaccination Requirements**
- **Other CDC-Recommended Immunizations**
- **Personnel Preferences or Allergies**

PATIENT/CLIENT PROTECTION

- **Comprehensive Medical History Evaluation and Patient's Oral Health Assessment to Facilitate the Treatment Plan**
- **Preprocedural Antiseptic Mouthrinse for the Patient**
- **Protective Barriers/Eyewear for the Patient**
- **Respiratory Hygiene and Cough Etiquette at www.cdc.gov/flu/professionals/infectioncontrol/resphygiene.htm**

PROVIDER/CLINICIAN ANTISEPSIS

- **Antiseptic Handwash as indicated**

PROVIDER/CLINICIAN BARRIERS

- Disposable Face Mask/Face Shield/Both
- Task-Appropriate Gloves
- Protective Eyewear
- Task-Appropriate Protective Attire

OPERATORY PROCESSING

- SOP for Environmental Surface Disinfection and the Use of Barriers
- Surface Cleaner/Tuberculocidal Disinfectant
- Surface/Equipment Barrier Protection
- Appropriate PPE

WASTE CONTAINMENT, MANAGEMENT, AND DISPOSAL

- Medical Waste Disposal System
- Waste Segregation
- Sharps Disposal System
- Appropriate Disposal of all Critical, Semicritical, and Noncritical Single-Use Items
- Appropriate PPE

ASEPTIC CONSIDERATIONS FOR CHAIRSIDE ASEPSIS

- Plan Procedural Needs
- Unit Dose
- Prevent Contamination
- Reduce Aerosolization
- Reduce Biofilm Release
- Wear Appropriate PPE

INSTRUMENT REPROCESSING SYSTEM

- Sterilize all Critical and Semicritical Reusable Items
- Wear Appropriate PPE
- Transport Contaminated Reusable Sharps in a Hard-Walled, Solid-Bottomed Container
- Presoak Items in a Holding Solution When Immediate Cleaning is not Possible
- Instrument Cleaning
- Package Items for Sterilization and Storage
- Utilize Only FDA-Cleared Sterilization Equipment
- Perform Sterilization Monitoring
- Perform Weekly Biologic Monitoring

INFECTION CONTROL CONSIDERATIONS FOR THE EXPOSURE AND PROCESSING OF RADIOGRAPHS

- Operatory Asepsis
- Processing Asepsis
- Appropriate PPE

INFECTION/EXPOSURE CONTROL IN THE LABORATORY AND IN THE OPERATORY WITH LABORATORY MATERIALS

- In-House Laboratory Policy and Procedures
- Outside Laboratory Infection Control Policies and Procedures for Transport/Handling
- Appropriate PPE

HAZARD COMMUNICATION

- Written Plan
- At-Risk Employees Identified
- Training
- Chemical Inventory
- SDS
- Emergency Equipment

POSTEXPOSURE MANAGEMENT AND FOLLOW-UP POLICY AND PROCEDURES

- Up-to-Date Confidential Employee Health Records
- Copies of the State and Federal Laws Regarding Patients' Rights, Issues of HIV Testing, and Confidentiality of Medical Information
- Injury/Incident Report Forms
- Workers' Compensation Forms
- Designated Healthcare Provider(s) for Postexposure Follow-up
- HIV Counseling and Testing Information
- Basic First Aid

COMMUNICATION OF HAZARDS

- Signs and Labels
- Posters

RECORD KEEPING

- Required
- Recommended

Discussion

Discuss with your Infection Control Coordinator or Safety Officer how the infection control and safety program is evaluated.

Notes